# Sleep, insomnia, stress: What you don't know can hurt you

### Patricia A. Farrell, Ph.D.

# ACKNOWLEDGMENTS

Books, as anyone who has ever written one or even attempted to write one, will tell you, do not write themselves and we all wish, at sometimes, they would. But, aside from the ideas and the research and writing, there are those who patiently make this journey with us and, in so doing, shepherd the task along.

I would be remiss if I did not thank members of my family who are still with us as well as those who have gone on to a much-deserved reward. Anyone who knows me will know to whom I refer, and their names shall remain inscribed in my heart forever. Thank you all for your love, understanding and tenacious loyalty through all the years we have been fortunate enough to have had together.

# PREFACE

The topic of sleep was something I took for granted like many of us. I knew people had problems sleeping, that insomnia was a common problem, sleep medications were being prescribed in increasing numbers and that there were many sleep disorders. But it wasn't until I became involved in a special sleep project years ago that my eyes were opened to what a major area this is and that consumers needed more information. Thus, I decided that I'd use my knowledge from the many meetings and conferences I attended to write this book.

As you read, there's one thing I think you should consider. This book isn't one you necessarily need to read straight through from beginning to end, but one where you can skip around to areas of interest. I've written it that way and that's the reason for the large reference section. References are where you can gather additional information you may find interests you or meets your needs, whatever they may be.

The intent here, also, is not to be an all-inclusive textbook, but a beginning for readers to understand more about sleep, the intricacies of what happens while we sleep and the seriousness of sleep. No longer, for me or you the reader, is sleep something that we do each day without knowing what I see as the magic that happens as we sleep. Also, it is interesting how we share so many sleep-related activities with birds, of all things, and how sleep plays an integral part in our physical and mental health. Sleep is literally a matter of life and death or impaired physical and mental health.

Saying that lack of sleep is something all of us must endure in this go-go world of ours is much too cavalier. We either sleep adequately or we give ourselves over to serious medical illnesses such as immune disorders, e.g., diabetes, work dysfunction and even death. Yes, sleep is that serious and not to be taken lightly.

With these thoughts in mind, I hope you find this book helpful in your efforts to improve your sleep, increase your joy in life and your creativity and approach sleep with the appreciation it truly deserves.

# TABLE OF CONTENTS

# CHAPTER 1

# why do we sleep?

◆ ◆ ◆

*The woods are lovely, dark and deep.*
*But I have promises to keep,*
*and miles to go before I sleep. -Robert Frost*

Sleep is one of the most powerful "medications" under your control plus it is nonprescription and extremely vital to every aspect of your life. In this book you will learn about the wonders of sleep and what it does for you. Be prepared for the ride because it's going to be incredibly exciting.

You will be introduced to new discoveries about sleep which have revealed it as one of the most potent forces in your body, regulating things you never dreamed about. You will increase not just your knowledge of sleep as a dire necessity, but the structures involved in sleep. No, it's not complicated but there are new words which you will utilize in the future as you progress in your understanding of what makes us want to sleep, what makes us go to sleep and what happens while we sleep.

Sleep isn't the quiet time you may have imagined. Actually, it's a time when your brain goes into overdrive to prepare for the next day. Additionally, it's tune-up time for the brain after the day you've just had. You may sleep, but your brain doesn't. Get the correct amount of sleep and you'll soon see it's part of maintaining a healthy lifestyle to manage your life and your future health.

Sleep is a natural part of all of our lives, yet we continue to wonder why we need to sleep. Today's world requires that we be not only awake and active for much of the time, but that we deny ourselves sleep. It appears that sleep has become something considered to be an inconvenience and a disruption of the normal life/work cycle expected of us. Is this true? Do we really not require sleep? Can we get by on three or four hours of sleep a night? Do we need to sleep at all?

Questions such as these require answers that are backed by scientific research and, from all of the research we have gathered over the past several decades, sleep is an absolutely essential part of a normal existence.

Without sleep, life would become not only impossible, but chaotic and bordering on psychiatric disorders. Lack of sleep would lead to our death. Yes, not sleeping can result in our dying prematurely or acting irrationally and taking our own life. Studies have shown this to be true.

The research does not indicate that not sleeping adequately results in death, but it can cause multiple physical and mental difficulties, and any reduction in the necessary number of hours of sleep is detrimental to us. The effects are on our immune system, our mental capacity to work and be creative and may predispose us to diseases such as cancer and diabetes and even obesity, not a disease but a serious problem.

Discoveries have indicated a paramount role of sleep in learning, memory, high blood pressure, diabetes, mood disorders, immune system disorders, dementia and behavioral problems in kids that can lead to suicide. In fact, sleep and suicide are two important factors currently upsetting school curriculums.

## The brain begins to reveal its secrets

Medical science had believed that the brain possessed just two "plumbing" systems that brought nourishment as well as necessary biological chemical elements to it. These two systems were important in removing toxins and bathing the brain in fluid. Together the systems provided a level of nutrition and safety against injury while removing waste materials.

In other words, the brain's connections were hooked up to the blood or circulatory system and the cerebrospinal fluid system (the CNS) and that was the total of its hook-ups. But scientists were totally unaware of the yet-to-be-discovered connection to the lymphatic system. The lymphatic system is the somewhat free-flowing and open fluid system in the body used by the immune system to carry its warrior white blood cells to battle disease.

The lymphatics are, as you may know, also the cleaners of the body. They are the first part of our body to warn of infection, inflammation and disease. Got a blister and notice that fluid in it? That's part lymph from our white blood cells working to stop an infection. And they are particularly vital when it comes to brain cleaning.

But who knew this system was involved in cleaning out the brain? Who considered that the brain needed cleaning each night? It never entered the minds of scientists studying brain pathology, so how could we be expected to give that particular bodily function a thought? Sleep was a period of rest, nothing more, or so scientists thought.

Lymphatics, as I've indicated, are also actively involved in carrying vital killer white cells (our warrior cells) to fight what they perceive as dangerous foreign tissue from virus/bacteria. The cells attack cancer and are being utilized in therapies for that disease. These are the cells that sometimes also fail to recognize "good" from "bad" materials and try to kill off donor organs in the body.

When this happens, it's one time when our beloved lymphatics are used, much to our dismay, in a nefarious way. These cells in the immune system may be involved in *disease initiation*.

"Clever" malignant cells can trick the immune system into doing the exact opposite of what their specific function is; protecting us from disease. Instead of helping, they start killing. When this happens, we're usually looking at an autoimmune disorder and there are many of them around.

## Brain cleaning during sleep

The cerebrospinal fluid system (the CNS) bathing the brain was believed to be the only brain lymphatic clean-up/maintenance hook-up. But then scientists discovered a new connection. A new name also had to be derived for this new system, so they put a brain cell name (the glial cells) together with the lymphatics and came up with *the glymphatic system*. More on that in *Chapter 2*.

## Sleep rewires the brain

Recent research using high resolution 3D brain scans (Vivo et al., 2017) revealed just how beneficial sleep is for our brains. They referred to what happens in the brain as "synaptic remodeling" or rewiring because it's actively adding to connections.

Over a four-year span, investigators at several research sites actually viewed how brain synapses, those tiny nerve connections, decrease in size during sleep. They decrease about 12-18% in size and the researchers theorize that this is more evidence for brain cleaning and rejuvenation activity during sleep. The action has been compared to a sponge being wrung out to release fluid, but here it's brain tissue and *it's doing this on its own.* It's also opening wider gaps between cells to aid the flushing action along and help get the toxin cleared from the brain.

But there is also another idea here regarding those powerful brain synapses and that is that they need to "recalculate" during sleep. You could say it's a means of brain recalibrating just as your car's GPS spurts out "recalculating" when you've made a wrong turn or computer hard drives need to defrag. Many activities in our body reflect computers, in fact.

The bottom line is that the brain is performing sleep-related functions to assist in daytime activity. Not all synapses seem to be involved in this sleep shrinkage task and larger, stronger ones may be left untouched in order to preserve memory.

Researchers also found that there might be a reason for sleepiness, too, and that was the work of a specific protein (Homer1a) that brought on sleepiness. The protein then promoted sleep and the brain got to work, but one thing interfered with the protein's action. What was it? Caffeine. Yes, that cup of coffee does its work on this sleep-promoting protein and prevents it from doing its job; getting us to sleep.

But what about brain clearing in addition to synaptic wiring changes? Knowledge about this vital pathway for clearing metabolic waste from the brain was further expanded to include yet another factor: *sleep posture.* Posture has an effect on the efficacy of this subtle system brain-cleaning system as we sleep and it's an important factor when you consider the alternative.

Using imaging, it was determined that both the supine and lateral (sleeping on your side) positions actually facilitated the brain clearing. Sleep position, therefore, plays another vital role in the action needed to protect you and your precious brain from waste accumulation.

Want to help the cleaners? Sleep on your side and you'll be doing just that. A researcher theorized that, although the actual reason for this positioning being optimal wasn't apparent, it was most probably due to some artifact of evolution.

Darwin had it right, then, when he said that evolution depended on the survival of the fittest. If we apply that idea to sleep and positioning, it would mean that our forebears who slept on their sides lived longer to reproduce because they were able to quickly and cleverly escape predators. They had clearer brains. Right? So, the tendency to sleep on your side is, in fact, an evolutionary wiring component of our species which promotes survival.

Which side should you sleep on, according to research? The *left side* appears to be the better side for brain cleaning. They offered no answer regarding why this side is better, but their imaging studies did show a decided difference here. We are left wondering, unfortunately.

But it may be a function of those ancestors who survived did sleep on their left side rather than their right. In fact, it may have something to do with which hand is dominant in defending against a threat. The usual hand would be the right hand, so sleeping on the left side would leave this hand free to grab a weapon.

## Sleep and brain health

Besides brain cleaning, there's an internal mechanism which puts us on a schedule. This *biological or circadian clock*, which regulates everything in our life has now been given more importance. This "clock" divides our 24-hour days into times for eating, digesting food, sleep and avoiding predators. Today, of course, we have little evidence that we need to protect ourselves from predators, but these structures are still present and still active in our brains. Surprisingly, two different areas of the brain are still functioning with those ancient predators in mind and we'll discuss that later in the book.

This "master clock," known to scientists as the suprachiasmatic nucleus (SCN), is located in an area of the brain called the hypothalamus. Its functions include checking the light in our environment plus the temperature and feeding time to adapt our behaviors to appropriate periods of the day or night. Knowing about this specialized biological clock has opened up new realizations regarding the role of sleep and health. Going against this natural clock is now seen as the culprit in matters of health.

One discovery was made more than two decades ago but it's only now that the non-scientific community is hearing about it. Since that time, it had not received the attention it deserved until recently. The scientist who made this breakthrough, Dr. Joseph S. Takahashi, published a revolutionary paper related to his discovery.

Circadian rhythms, as you just discovered, are vital to our existence but there is an assumption that had been questioned by Dr..Takahashi, of the UT Southwestern Medical Center in Dallas, Texas. Over 25 years ago, this scientist noticed something truly groundbreaking and it *wasn't confined to the brain.*

Ask yourself a question. Where do you think our circadian "clock" would be in our bodies? Probably your answer would be that it has to be in the brain since it is so involved in sleep and waking. The assumption, according to Dr. Takahashi's research, would be inaccurate. He has discovered what is known as the *CLOCK gene* which controls circadian rhythms or our biological clock. This gene is *in every cell in our bodies.*

In fact, the cells in the skin, i.e., CLOCK genes, are responsible for protecting us against the ultraviolet rays of the sun and, therefore, warding off skin cancer. Cancer, in fact, has been found to be higher in night shiftworkers. Researchers are interested in determining if a problem in our circadian rhythm occurs due to night shiftwork and non-exposure to sunshine. If that is the case, then working nights could be detrimental to people's health. And, as you learn later The World Health Organization has stated that night shiftwork is a *probable cause of cancer.*

Not only is the CLOCK gene involved in cancer, it may also be involved in dieting and in determining the best time of day to eat. Eating at the wrong time at night, according to Dr. Takahashi's research, will not lead to weight loss even while you're dieting. The fact is that timing our eating is essential since metabolism is highly regulated by the CLOCK gene. And, as we sleep, this gene provides direction to our utilization of the byproducts of metabolism to prepare for the next day.

Dieting and food consumption isn't the only issue. The CLOCK gene is believed to have an impact on our lifespan and longevity. The implications for this research finding are far-reaching with incredible future promise. Now that we know more about this unique gene, the thinking is that it acts much like a conductor directing a finely tuned orchestra in the sonata of life. Everything appears to follow the lead of this pervasive gene and its importance cannot be underscored too strongly.

The effects of this work are now more fully understood and fresh new insights mean new breakthroughs in areas of mental and physical health. One question which requires answering is whether there is a definite, probably genetic, relationship to health and your being a "lark" or an "owl." See our *Appendix B* to take a short test.

Is this related to your CLOCK gene and particular type of daytime or nighttime functioning? Would it determine whether you are, biologically, better suited to working days or nights? Should *careers or work environments* be centered around your particular CLOCK gene's orientation? Interesting questions.

Another question that still remains to be tackled is whether sleep deprivation and disruption of the circadian clock causes health damage. Or is it disease that disrupts sleep and then there's a feedback loop that deepens this health quandary? How does the CLOCK gene fit into this and *can it be reprogrammed* in some way? A classic question of which came first, the "chicken or the egg?" For us, it's yet another mystery the brain and the body have not allowed us to solve and which remains for future researchers to unravel.

## Sleep myths

What do we now believe about sleep? Probably the great majority of us knew nothing about the CLOCK gene but we do hold strong beliefs about sleep. Eager to tackle that one, a group of scientists began scouring the internet for answers.

What about the myth that people can get by with sleeping less than five hours a night and there's no effect on their physical and mental health? A recent study at New York University of 8,000 websites looked at the 20 most popular sleep myths.

The researchers concluded that getting less than seven hours of sleep a night is likely to result in deficits in cardiovascular functioning and metabolic risks which are associated with diabetes. There are also mental and immune disorder problems that are associated with insufficient sleep. But the thinking still persists that we can function find on less sleep.

One of the primary purposes of their research study was to begin to help the public to change their thinking about sleep and that you can't get by on less sleep and still function well. The conclusion was that this is an *absolute myth* which has absolute serious consequences. They note that among the myths they discovered on these websites were:

1. *Your brain can function without sleep* – it can't and while some people can adjust to less sleep, it does not mean their health will not suffer. Which would you pick, adequate sleep or *cancer*? How about adequate sleep or a *stroke*? Perhaps, *if you're a man*, adequate sleep or *inability to have children*?
2. *Lying in bed with your eyes closed is almost as good as sleeping*: the researchers indicate this is absolutely wrong since there are still problems in the endocrine, cardiovascular and metabolic activity during this wakefulness. These disruptions do not permit the person to go into what is known as REM sleep. An analogy by the researchers was that this was as effective as going to the gym and standing still on a treadmill.
3. *Exercise before bed* is still a topic where research is inconclusive, however, mild exercise such as yoga might be beneficial.
4. *Adults sleep less as they get older* – again, it's not clear if older adults do require less sleep than young adults. But we know there is a relationship between going to bed early (around 8-9PM) and awaking at 4-5AM with retirement and/or stress.

5. *Alcohol before bed can improve sleep* – research indicates that while this may get you to sleep, it disturbs the natural sleep cycle during the night. It will cause interruptions which may have long-term detrimental effects because of its interference with the natural cyclic waves we experience during sleep.

One of the conclusions the researchers did come to, after inspecting all of the websites, was that *sleep hygiene* did not receive enough attention on these websites and that was *a primary problem.*

Sleep hygiene, as has been discussed later in this book, is of crucial importance and is one of the best ways to promote healthy, restful sleep.

# CHAPTER 2

# The Brain and Sleep

◆ ◆ ◆

*Think in the morning.*
*Act in the noon.*
*Eat in the evening.*
*Sleep in the night. – William Blake*

Only recently have we discovered that the brain has been holding onto yet another of its sleep secrets. This latest secret of the brain has been revealed by delicate microscopic inspection of brain tissue. An incredible connection to one of the world's most important biological "waterways," in terms of the lymphatic system, was accidentally discovered. We introduced this earlier in *Chapter 1.*

## The discovery of the glymphatic system

The latest discovery in the brain cleaning/maintenance system is now known as the *glymphatic system* after the cells involved in it. The system had lain hidden in plain sight until curiosity struck a researcher who did further work with powerful microscopic equipment and there it was.

The upper regions of the pathway lead down the neck and go into the other portions of the body's lymphatic system and provides a conduit for the brain fluid there. How did the new system get its name? A simple combination of the major cells that hold brain cells together and provide other important functions (the *glial cells*) and the *lymphatic system*. Voila, a new system was born and named. Did we think there'd be any more brain secrets?

The value of this discovery can be more fully appreciated when we hear that this is a game changer. It is so important that it will require rewriting current medical textbooks on sleep and the brain. It has also opened up an entire new area of exploration of the sleeping brain and how it works.

## New Rose Hip brain cell discovered

After the discovery of the glymphatic system, another brain researcher found a previously unknown brain cell, the *Rose Hip cell*. These cells, shaped somewhat like a rose after the petals have fallen off, are believed to be involved in anxiety control, but no one knows for sure. They are, in fact, not found in mice, which means brain research with mice may be flawed. The future waits for yet more discoveries about this neuron and what the brain may still be hiding from us.

The frontier of brain science has, again, been pushed into new territory. The prospects, too, are exciting and not just in sleep research. New technology is coming into play and it provides new windows into the brain.

Recent research using high resolution 3D brain scans revealed just how beneficial sleep is for our brains. They referred to what happens in the brain as "synaptic remodeling." Remember, in Chapter 1 I made mention of "rewiring?"

Over a four-year span, investigators at several research sites actually viewed how brain synapses, the billions of brain connections that serve as information highways in the brain, *decrease in size during sleep*. They decrease about 12-18% in size and the researchers theorize that this is more evidence for brain cleaning and rejuvenation activity during sleep. How could the brain reduce in size during sleep and then return to its normal size when we wake up? We still need more information here.

The main point is that the brain is performing sleep-related functions to assist in daytime activity. Not all synapses seem to be involved in this sleep shrinkage task and larger, stronger ones may be left untouched in order to preserve memory. The mystery of which ones engage in size change and which do not has not been solved at this point but we will know in the not-too-distant future.

Do you know how active the sleeping brain is in fact? I'll bet that most people still think sleep is a quiet time for the brain to lull around in its cozy, warm environment and get a break.

The brain just kicks back and takes it easy, right? Well, that's far from the truth as we now know and it's a rather frantic time of activity. It's like Santa Clause's elves right before Christmas Eve.

## Sleep and brain shrinkage

When we go to sleep, the brain gets busy and, in fact, probably busier than ever. Cells that were once plump during the day as they worked to keep you functioning now do something unheard of—they shrink in size.

Yes, as you sleep as you now know, your brain is shrinking but it's a good thing, so don't get upset. As the cells shrink, channels between them open wider to allow for the passage of waste products of metabolism. It begins a flow to prepare for the coming day and it happens effortlessly, or so we think because we're off in dreamland.

Who knew that sleeping would actually change the configuration or size of the cells in the brain? You'll read later in this book about brain regions in adolescents and how they change as a function of sleep, which, in turn, affects how teens do academically.

Certainly, brain researchers weren't aware of it and they must have been scratching their heads. But I'll bet whoever discovered it was rubbing their hands in glee and jumping up in the air. It's a discovery worthy of a Nobel Prize.

## Brain weight and learning

Did you know that the only other time we already knew that the brain changed its size was when we learned something new? Researchers have known that learning results in heavier brains. Learning translates into the brain making more and stronger nerve connections (synapses) and the more you learn, theoretically, the stronger these connections and, at the same time, they bulk up. Not exactly like putting your brain on steroids, but it does what you want it to do; helps you learn and retain what you've learned provided you put that learning into long term memory (LTM).

The gym for this brain size increase, of course, is under your control as you read, watch and learn new things as well as going over things you learned in the past. In the latter, you do repair work on the neural highway to bring it up to speed again. Think of forgetting as a way for the brain to put material into cold storage. When you need it, a quick tune-up on the old material will bring it back.

Do we ever forget? Probably not but it may be difficult to access certain material we learned long ago. However, it's there.

Studying just prior to sleep or reading material you want to use later is your entrance to your own brain "gym" and you've got a six-pack that can only be seen on a CT scan. We know this from studies that have been done in research with learning and its effect on brain volume and weight.

No, don't worry. You won't get a fat head because there's still plenty of room inside your skull to accommodate this expansion of those neural nets. And, if you want to keep your brain in the best form it can be for as long as it can, *lifelong learning is the way to go*. Each new bit of learning adds to that precious reservoir of your brain and its memory banks which are most certainly physical in nature.

Exercising your brain, even while you sleep, is pretty easy when you think about it. Read prior to sleep and you will retain the information better than if you didn't read or study just before you went to sleep. Sleep, therefore, provides memory consolidation of information from short-term to long-term memory and this is especially helpful for students or workers wishing to remember important information.

Pulling all-nighters or cramming before an exam and denying yourself sleep is NOT a memory aid, however. Study, sleep and wake up to go over the material once again, rather than doing this in one prolonged all-night session.

## A "new" brain each morning

Remember one thing. *The brain you had when you went to sleep is not the brain you will have when you awaken in the morning*. It will have changed its configuration and for the better because *it is making those new connections as you sleep*. Sleep, therefore, is your most powerful means of learning and a brain repair mechanism you have under your control. *Yes, it's your control, not your teacher's, not your parents, not your boss, but YOU.*

But there's a contradiction here and that's okay. Why do the cells of your brain begin to shrink even as they grow and strengthen these new connections while you sleep? Doesn't that mean something is wrong with our brains when it begins to shrink?

We hear disturbing things about shrinking brains and then there's the belief about each martini you drink killing how many millions of brain cells? Makes you shudder, doesn't it? Sure, alcohol is a brain toxin, but there is hope here, too. Moderation is the key as it is to almost everything else.

And whenever we hear about shrinking brains, too, it's usually in terms of things like Alzheimer's and memory loss, right? Not good stuff. Oh, no, but there's still more.

Mysteries are being discovered as you sit and read about the sleeping brain. In fact, we know that the brain has a "bank account" of stem cells it can use when needed, so there may be more regeneration of brain cells going on than we know at this moment.

We've only heard about cell destruction, but apparently it may work both ways; cell destruction and cell creation. You may have heard the term neurogenesis. A specific substance, in fact, has been found to promote nerve growth and it's known as NGF (nerve growth factor).

Brain cells may be dying off and flushed away once they reach their life expectancy, but they may also be replaced and that offers a lot of hope to many people. When we consider new brain cells, we think of stem cells called "undifferentiated" cells. This type of cell has the potential for being formed into almost any type of cell that the body might need. Therefore, they are tiny miracles waiting to be called upon to go into action and provide replacement resources where needed.

Although you may know that stem cells are found in the bone marrow of your body, there are two places in the brain, the lateral ventricles (small open areas in the brain) and the hippocampus (the primary memory center of the brain) where they reside, too.

Unbelievably, our brain has a number of these discrete open spaces which provide a newly-discovered resource for stem cells that can be utilized in brain cell repair. The brain ventricles are filled with fluid, but they are also lined in a number of specific areas with these specialized cells lying dormant and waiting.

The task for future researchers, therefore, is to determine how best to access, stimulate, or utilize these cells in whatever manner is needed. Of course, this is the basis for what is known as stem cell therapy and future efforts will broaden its horizon beyond anything we can imagine today.

## The brain's repair mechanism

During sleep, it seems that the brain may be repairing itself with these specialized master cells and this introduces an entirely new perspective on sleep and its utility to us. Imagine that we can actually help our body repair itself by simply going to sleep. Can you think of anything that is simpler and at the same time more complex without any effort on your part? Sleep, as it were, is a "therapy" or a "medication" without any prescription other than that you get the sleep you need to facilitate this brain function.

The discovery of these stem cells in the brain and their ability to repair portions of the brain is one of many that have been made during this decade. We now know that the body, in addition to the brain, is still holding its secrets and there are yet more to be discovered. The potential must be incredibly exciting for new researchers entering the field because of the vastness of potential discoveries that awaits them.

Future scientists, undoubtedly, will be able to use this neural cell reservoir to treat a variety of brain-related illnesses. We do not know if during sleep any of them may be pressed into service, but it's comforting to know they are there. Imagine if we could cure Alzheimer's (Senile Dementia of the Alzheimer's Type or SDAT) by making a withdrawal from this brain bank to repopulate brain areas destroyed by SDAT or Parkinson's Disease or other neurological disorders or even stroke?

The prospect of finding a "cure" for SDAT is very exciting because it is viewed as the scourge of older individuals and it can't be ignored. The coming decades will see an ever-increasing number of persons with SDAT which will place an incredible financial burden on families and countries in terms of care for these individuals.

## Brain cell loss?

Are we losing our brain cells as we sleep and is that the "shrinking" I'm describing? No, that's not what I'm writing about here. Simply put, the thinking is that the brain cells are pushing out all the trash of the day (trash meaning metabolic waste from all that daily brain activity) into that newly-discovered lymph system so it can be swept away. The cells of the brain are filled with "trash" and it must be, literally, wrung out because it can't hold more.

If you don't let it clean up, what will happen? We know that some of that waste material is from specific material, called *tau*, which provides helpful functioning to nerve cells but also breaks down. Tau can then be involved in cell destruction that we see in Alzheimer's. Once this happens and it accumulates and isn't eliminated, the danger begins, so it is vital that the "cleaners" get to work as you slumber.

Think of all the activity that your brain is required to engage in during your waking hours and you may foster a new appreciation of how vital the cleaning process (aka sleep) is. Not only does the brain allow you to think, plan, move your limbs, send messages to various organs to function properly, keep your heart beating and your lungs working, it has too many activities to even recount adequately here. The brain is a super activated organ or, perhaps, a combination organ/gland.

The brain isn't just busy during your waking hours, it is incredibly overburdened with multi-tasking and every single one of those actions produces a vast amount of waste material in the brain. All of that "garbage" needs to be discarded quickly and efficiently or you will suffer the consequences.

If the debris weren't discarded, most probably, you would quickly fail to function in countless ways. Not sleeping is tantamount to not taking out the garbage and just allowing it to accumulate in your kitchen until you are shoulder deep in it and cannot move. Pretty horrible thought, right? Yes, it is.

The change in brain cell size was first observed in laboratories studying mice but it applies to we humans as well. This cell cleaning and shrinking seems to be implicated in the *sleep duration of specific animals*, us included. In fact, it seems likely that's the reason infants need to sleep longer than adults; different brain sizes require more or less hours of cleaning. And, the growth years of children involve an abundance of neural growth and connections as new ones are formed and old connections may die off. Thus, the reason kids need more sleep.

## Brain cleaning during sleep

Sleep, it appears therefore, is directly related to brain size and the brain's ability to accumulate and store toxic leftovers from daily activity. Another of these toxic leftovers may be the deadly beta amyloid and resultant plaques thought to be involved in the development of Alzheimer's and other brain disorders.

If this amyloid, just like tau, could be efficiently and swiftly expelled from brain cells to keep them from dying, might we also conquer some types of Alzheimer's? Very tempting thought there.

Have you ever given any thought to why babies sleep so much or how much puppies sleep? The researchers believe it's because of their brain size and the toxic build-up in brain cells that necessitates cleaning and that can *only be accomplished* during sleep.

Remember, babies and puppies share something in common; both of them are on an incredible new-learning adventure. The amount of information that they are acquiring daily is extraordinary, but they have small brains. Smaller brains=more time needed for sleep-cleaning.

Makes sense, doesn't it? Smaller brains can hold *less* toxins, so they need more downtime to clean up and get ready for action again. So, sleep and getting cleaned up is the ticket for the brain.

During sleep the brain it's time for the cleaners to come in and dump all those wastebaskets out and leave the place fresh for another day of activity. If you prevent the cleaners from doing their job, as I've already said, you are placing yourself at great risk, possibly even greater risk than you ever imagined. And it's just a simple matter of sleep, something over which you DO have quite a bit of control in many cases.

Of course, we wonder if naps are also a "cleaning up" time for the brain and that's why our body's natural circadian rhythm (our body clock) puts us into that desire for an afternoon nap. After all, if sleep can clean the brain, why wouldn't a nap do the same? Power nap, indeed. It's sort of your little cleaning machine doing a job.

# CHAPTER 3

# The Stages of Sleep

◆ ◆ ◆

*Sleep is the best meditation – Dalai Lama*

Sleep isn't simply a time when we doze off and go into a wonderful state of rest, restoration and memory consolidation, as you've already read. It's a period of time when our brain also exhibits a *fluctuating rhythm of electronic waves* and there are stages of sleep. Each stage is controlled autonomously by the brain, not us.

We go from light to deep sleep with resultant changes in our breathing, heart rates and body temperature. It is also a time of dreaming, sometimes intentional and often without any effort on our part. The major muscles of the body, too, may become paralyzed, perhaps helping to maintain movement to assist us in maintaining our sleep.

## Stage 1:

A light sleep stage where there may be some muscle twitching. Only 4-5% of sleep of the whole sleep cycle will be spent here. It is often referred to as light sleep and we can be awakened quite easily. During this time there may be sudden, unexpected muscle contractions known as hypnic jerks or hypnic myoclonia and people will often say they had the sensation of starting to fall. Some people do fall out of bed.

### Stage 2:

A slowing of both breathing and heart rates and a decrease in body temperature. About 45-55% of the whole cycle is spent in this stage. This is where eye muscles stop moving, brainwave activity becomes slower and, if we were to hook someone up to electrodes, we would see that there were brainwave bursts called *sleep spindles*.

### Stage 3:

Deep sleep begins. Again, there is a slowing of the brain waves called Delta waves and it is at this time during Stages 3 and 4 that it would be difficult to awaken someone

### Stage 4:

Often grouped together with Stage 3, this is when the deep sleep stage begins with another change in brain wave activity, limited or paralyzed muscle activity and rhythmic breathing is apparent.

### Stage 5 (REM Sleep):

Often not referred to as a stage of sleep, this is one of the most active and important times during your sleep cycle. In this sleep period, the dreaming stage begins, with some uptick in heart rate and rapid, shallow breathing. REM sleep is a period during which muscles are temporarily paralyzed. This period begins between 70 – 90 minutes after we fall asleep. Most people will spend much of their sleep time in Stages 1, 2, and REM.

REM (Rapid Eye Movement), as you may know, occurs at those times when you would think we'd be in the deepest sleep. Oddly, this isn't the case. Just prior to awakening, you experience this dreaming state and perhaps that's why you remember those dreams, but to what are they related?

Some dreams are available to your memory and some aren't. Why is this? Good questions but not with good answers at this stage of the research. We don't know if dreams are figments of what is happening in our environment at the moment or just a function of our brain trying to put some sense to the cleaning activity that is occurring.

The discovery of the stages of sleep then led to further exploration of the fundamentals of sleep and its biochemistry. What was the essential life role not only related to our psychological well-being but our physical health as well that sleep played? The researchers didn't know it then, but there are very real physical disorders connected to sleep and sleep deprivation (aka *sleep debt*) disorders.

Prior to Dr. Nathaniel Kleitman's work, sleep was a mysterious condition of semi-consciousness that was treated as a somewhat mystical state, a time that provided portends for the future. It was for Freud the "royal road to the unconscious" and something that required analysis rather than biological exploration.

Dreaming was fodder for interpretation. Now we know that dreams come from many things such as the environment where we're sleeping, concerns of the day and actions of the brain cleaning out the clutter or "code" of the day to put it in computer terms.

Cleaning always involves some degree of drama in the brain, it seems. But it seems dreams can also be "programmed" to help us answer questions we have and this activity has fascinating potential which we explore in *Chapter 14*.

If the brain functions much like a biological computer, it may require defragging and sleep could be the time when this program is put into action. You're the programmer here even if you don't know how to code. The brain does it for you if you allow it. It makes sense that this "machine" needs to reposition information, too, in order to help us with our memory for the next day.

Each sleep stage has a function but there is still much to be learned regarding sleep, the stages of sleep and the damage that sleep deprivation can wreak. The final frontier may not only be in the brain but in its sleep activity as well.

# CHAPTER 4

# Are You a Lark or an Owl?

◆ ◆ ◆

*Though sleep is called our best friend, it is a friend*
*who often keeps us waiting! – Jules Verne*

Sleep research has now identified two major distinct types of what is known as circadian rhythm or chronobiology, the body's internal clock that establishes sleep preference and waking performance for us. These innate rhythms set our sleep and wake times for us and they may be able to be changed. In fact, as we age, our sleep patterns change, too.

The two major categories of chronotypes are:

## 1. The Lark: Early to bed

The lark is the person who when daylight saving time comes around, may need to know one thing; lark or owl (Sheikh, 2016)? Highly different styles of tucking in for the night and awakening in the morning exist for each type of sleeper.

Larks tend to go to bed earlier, while owls stay up late and have problems getting up in the morning. Larks, on the other hand, arise ready for the day and breakfast. BTW, it's pretty much genetically determined and, as we get older, more of us will turn into larks.

The "lark" and the "owl" determination is helpful. Here's a link to a self-report questionnaire from the Ludwig-Maximilians-Universitat Munchen and you'll find it here: http://bitly.com/2lVdOvl. We've also included a test in *Appendix B*.

If you are a shiftworker, they're working on a variation of the test for you. Until then though you might want to see if you are a lark or an owl and why that might be a problem for you with your schedule.

## 2. The Owl: Late to bed

Owls, as we know from those lovely winged creatures, come out at night and that's when they function, so anyone who is an "owl" here does best at night, not in the morning.

Each of the two, and there might be more, who knows, are determined by our body's own internal clock, highly dependent on your genetic inheritance. Later in life, however, nature may swing you out of that owl phase and into more of an early, early lark phase when you awaken at 4 a.m. in the morning.

Chronotype, which is a person's preferred sleep timing, and their work schedule was investigated to see if there was a relationship between sleep and Type II diabetes risk.

## A study of nurses and larks/owls

A study of nurses followed 64,000 women over a six-year period in what is known as early chronotypes (the Larks). The risk of Type II diabetes was associated with the duration of the shiftwork. Late chronotypes (the Owls) had the *highest diabetes risk when they worked daytime shifts*. The study, as the researchers saw it, indicated that work shifts should be timed with an individual's chronotype.

But nurses also are in a profession where stress is high, job support is insufficient, burnout is not addressed, and suicide is an issue not to be spoken of even on the unit. Therefore, regardless of whether they are larks or owls, they do lose sleep because of shift changes and demands.

Numerous laboratory studies have shown that sleep loss can be associated with glucose metabolism and insulin and, therefore, with developing Type II diabetes. The Owls exhibited higher blood A1c (glucose) levels and appeared to be at higher risk for diabetes metabolic syndrome.

Now, how about asking yourself a few questions about how you've been feeling lately? This is just to provide you with some additional information about where you might want to make some changes.

# How have you been sleeping?

Number of hours you sleep: _____
Have you been having conflicts with anyone?          ___yes ___no
Do you find yourself becoming anxious?               ___yes ___no
Do you feel you have little time for yourself?       ___yes ___no
Are you feeling depressed?                           ___yes ___no
Do you feel trapped in any way?                      ___yes ___no
Is a sense of resentfulness taking over you?         ___yes ___no

There's no score for these last few questions but in thinking each of them over, you may begin to come in touch with things that are bothering you. If you're not sleeping well, what might be the reason? What about having conflicts with anyone? Is this something new for you? How often is it happening? Are you finding that you are short-tempered? Do little things bother you more than they used to? Sleep deprivation can have a dramatic effect on all of these and that may be the culprit.

What about your level of anxiety? Everyone gets anxious sometime and that's normal because there are things that make all of us anxious. But if you're feeling more anxious than usual, what is the source of that anxiety? Might it be that you feel you're not up to the demands of what you have to do in your life and you're just feeling exhausted by everything? Think it over.

If you bought this book in paperback or e-book, feel free to mark it up, put notes in anywhere, underline, do whatever and highlight if possible—anything that will help you to utilize it more fully. And don't forget that reading once is often not sufficient to retain information. Reread what you've already read so that you reinforce your information. No, there are no quizzes here, but you will benefit by keeping your information on sleep fresh in your memory banks.

Need I add an additional word about allowing yourself the pleasure and restoration you need by sleeping or napping when you can, as much as you can? I'm not advocating that you engage in a life of total leisure here, but I want you to give yourself a break; you deserve it.

Workers are at their most creative when they have adequate sleep. No one is doubting that even when billionaire inventors are suggesting otherwise. There is no escape from the need for sleep. Thinking otherwise is dangerous. If you have one life to live, don't you want it to be the best one you can possibly have? Sleep is one answer.

I have to wonder how much damage is done to workers who are led to believe that working all night long on a project and not getting adequate sleep is okay. It may not be readily apparent this week or this month, but somewhere down the line, there will be a price to pay and who can repay you for lost health?

I know how hard all of you work at your many roles and each takes something from you, so be sure to recharge those emotional and physical batteries and don't skimp on sleep.

# CHAPTER 5

# OK, What About Sleep Myths?

◆ ◆ ◆

*Sleeping is no mean art: for its sake*
*one must stay awake all day. -Friedrich Nietzsche*

Sleep myths still exist in various parts of the world and some of the beliefs are so strong that they can result in death. For instance, have you ever heard of "ghost death" or as it is sometimes referred to as "nightmare death?" There is a belief in Asia about terrifying dreams that are, in fact, so terrifying that they kill.

Was it a terrifying dream that caused their deaths while they slept? One pathologist believes it is stress related and that their hearts just gave out while they slept and a frightening dream may have been the precipitant. But they were also in unfamiliar and possibly dangerous surrounding that would have caused surges in stress hormones, and that could have triggered pre-existing heart problems.

## Beauty Sleep

Is it true that sleep can have an effect on your facial appearance and is there such a thing as "beauty sleep?" Apparently, there is a relationship between the attractiveness that others find in us and whether or not we've had enough sleep, or we look tired. It seems that those who are sleepy have decreased attractiveness and health according to others viewing them.

Research has indicated that not only are we seen as collectively less attractive, but people are less inclined to want to interact with us socially and we are seen as less healthy and sleepier. Sleep loss, they indicated, is apparent in our facial appearance and that is the secret that everyone needs to know because sleep does have an effect on how beautiful we may be perceived. In addition, lack of sleep makes us perceive things in a negative manner and that colors our relationships.

Medical professionals, specifically dermatologists who deal with skin issues, have indicated that as we sleep the skin makes vital new collagen that prevents skin sagging. It's considered an important repair process and results in skin that is plumper and less likely to wrinkle. Persons who received five hours or less a night, were seen by these professionals as having twice as many fine lines on their face as those who got at least seven hours.

Less sleep also results in drier skin which makes those wrinkles more visible. Additionally, sleep promotes increased blood flow in the skin, especially of the face, which can result in a healthier coloration and enhance the complexion so that it doesn't look drab or ashen.

What else can sleep do to increase our attractiveness? Dark circles under the eyes are a result of inadequate sleep as is the puffiness around the eyes we often see. Want less puffiness and less tendency to develop dark circles? Sleep is the beauty answer because it provides moisture to your skin.

The dark circles, in fact, are an indication that the blood in the skin of the face may not be flowing as well as it might, and it can collect under the eyes where the skin is thinnest. Of course, circles under the eyes are also affected by your genetic inheritance, your age and even the pigment in your skin that is natural in your family.

Apart from the skin, sleep helps maintain healthy hair, possibly preventing breakage and damage which appears to be a result of inadequate nutrients reaching the scalp and providing less food, as it were, to this area. Of course, the stress of less sleep also means higher stress hormone levels which increases hair loss.

One additional consideration related to maintaining a healthy, youthful facial experience is that the skin can dry out more readily as we sleep and it is important to apply a moisturizer before going to sleep. Both men and women would benefit from this.

Aside from attractiveness, those who ensure adequate sleep each night are, according to research, more employable, seen as trustworthy, more intelligent and generally friendlier.

## The oracle of Delphi

Ancient Greeks believed in dream interpretation and the Oracle of Delphi who, while in a trance or sleep-like state, would provide answers to questions they posed. Was the trance a state of wakeful sleep? Who can tell us?

She was regarded as the ultimate authority and supplicants had to make their way up a mountain path and then into a series of chambers constructed to create a surreal experience. This method of creating another-world experience out of darkened chambers and pots of metal shavings was used by the physician Anton Mesmer in the nineteenth century when he devised the concept of animal magnetism or mesmerism, later known as hypnosis.

The Oracle of Delphi created a template of sorts, it would seem, for others who would wish to change reality in some fashion. Perceptual distortions could then be used in that newly created "reality" for some specific purpose.

Once in the presence of the Oracle, I'm sure the travelers were exhausted, lacked sleep and in an altered state of consciousness of their own.

## Present day "dreaming"

Reading about the Oracle, I couldn't help but be struck by the similarity between this journey and one that was required of everyone who went to psychiatrist Dr. Milton H. Erickson for training.

What type of training? Hypnosis, another altered state of consciousness, or so it is believed. Erickson had a unique induction he had developed over the years as a result of early polio that had left him almost totally paralyzed and in a wheelchair.

Erickson's method, which remains a subject of controversy, has proven sufficiently useful in some areas and attracts many professionals for train-ing. What was the lynchpin of his method? Metaphor. Wasn't that what the Oracle used, too, when proffering advice in the form of riddles or poems or even dreams?

Everyone who went for Ericksonian training with Dr. Erickson had to climb Camelback Mountain in the Arizona mountains as part of their learn-ing process.

They were told that when they got to the top they would discover some-thing. What that "something" was Erickson never told them. Each had to discover it for themselves, just as in a rare video recording (on YouTube) he told professionals they would have to discover their own techniques for themselves. Erickson died in 1980.

A form of self-hypnosis happens to all of us and we never realize that it's an altered state of consciousness with our eyes open—rather like sea-birds that sleep with open eyes. Know when it happens? During overly learned trips such as daily commuter trips where we remember getting into the car, train or bus and out of it but everything in between is a blank to us.

## Ancient Greek beliefs

The temples were places where people hoped to receive interpretation of their dreams. But, occasionally, they wished to be placed in "near-death" states for relief from their psychological and physical suffering. In other words, a type of sleep which would provide escape from their pain.

In some cases, induced dream states were used for simple surgical pro-cedures. It was believed that dreams, in fact, were indications of symptoms of disease and that interpreting them led to cures. Some dreams were sent by the gods and some sent by the soul. Each provided fruit for thought and exploration in terms of health.

## Ghost death

Sleep myths still exist in various parts of the world and some of the beliefs are so strong that they can result in death. For instance, "nightmare death." There is a belief in Asia about terrifying dreams that are, in fact, so terrify-ing that they kill.

Generally, "ghost death" happens to healthy young men in their middle 30s with no known similarities other than that they were refugees. Ghost deaths occur primarily in the Philippines (bangungut), Japan (pokkuri) and Thailand but may be found in the United States where these men have settled.

# CHAPTER 6

# The Man Who "Discovered" Sleep Medicine

◆ ◆ ◆

*We are such stuff as dreams are made on; and our little*
*life is rounded with a sleep.- William Shakespeare*

The question regarding how much we should sleep or why we need to sleep at all has been partially answered by research over the past several decades. Until Dr. Nathaniel Kleitman began researching the subject in the early part of the 19th Century, sleep was seen as ordinary and not requiring scientific exploration.

Time for a bit of history on sleep disorders just to fill you in on its past, its present state as sleep medicine and, possibly the future. One of the first books on sleep as a physical disorder was written in Europe in 1913 in France by Henri Pieron.

It was not until the 1920s that work was begun in earnest in Chicago, Illinois, USA by Dr. Nathaniel Kleitman the researcher who discovered one of the most important stages of sleep, REM. The discovery led to the development of the stages of sleep and that was the discovery that revealed what we now know as REM (rapid eye movement) sleep today.

Once REM was seen as signaling a specific stage of sleep, where active dreaming took place, the researchers began to look at sleep in terms of cycles or stages (five in all) rather than just one continuous sleep stage.

What we must remember is that most of our dreaming may occur just before we wake up but that doesn't mean we'll always remember our dreams.

Dreams have a fickle quality and may fade quickly with each waking moment. Should you be concerned? Not unless it is a disturbing, recurrent dream. Perhaps that might be an indication of something that needs your attention.

## History of sleep medicine

Sleep disorders, except for one or two, were not adequately categorized and remained largely unknown until Dr. Kleitman began delving into its mysteries. Once sleep research began in earnest, there was a new appreciation for how sophisticated this body mechanism was, and researchers vigorously considered an apparently new and largely unknown number of sleep disorders.

After Kleitman had performed the initial research experiments, one of his most brilliant students, Dr. William C. Dement, formally of California's Stanford University, involved himself in further extensive research. Dement produced one of the first books for the general public, "*Some Must Watch While Some Must Sleep.*"

The book provided new comprehension by a lay audience interested in understanding why they were having problems sleeping and what they might be able to do about it. It was a revelation for all those who were wondering both why they needed to sleep at all as well as why they couldn't sleep and were questioning how much sleep they needed.

To date, there are about 84 recognized sleep disorders separated into six different categories. It is estimated that sleep disorders account for approximately $70 billion annually in lost productivity, medical bills and industrial accidents. Sleep, as you can see, has risen as a serious concern with far-reaching consequences. Laughing it off is no longer a laughing matter and is a foolish endeavor.

One extremely unusual sleep disorder, which runs in families, *is Fatal Familial Insomnia (FFI)*. This form of insomnia results in death. If you wish to understand this better, there is a YouTube video, entitled "Dying to Sleep," which deals with FFI. Characteristics of this disorder include increasing insomnia but there are also hallucinations (for about five months), a complete inability to sleep, rapid weight loss (for about three months) and the final stage is death.

The course of the disorder is quite short. A word of caution is advisable here. Because you may have some of these symptoms doesn't mean that you have FFI, so please don't jump to conclusions. The disorder is *very rare*.

The number of sleep disorders currently is quite large, but we generally think only about one primarily and that one disorder is called *simple insomnia*. Insomnia is the inability to fall into deep, restful sleep. It can be episodic or prolonged. When it is prolonged, the consequences of this lack of restful sleep have only recently come to the fore and are now receiving serious medical attention.

Even the scientists and physicians working in the new burgeoning field of sleep medicine didn't know what they were in for and they were astonished as they unraveled the mysteries of sleep. Their dismay could only be matched by the relief of patients who had previously received a misdiagnosis with less-than-helpful treatments. Some patients were told they had a serious psychiatric disorder and treated for it. Others were left wondering what they had and who could help them. But first researchers had to embark on a journey into the recesses of the brain and the dark kingdom of the night.

Today, the discussion continues and the US Centers for Disease Control (CDC) indicates that, despite all the consumer education that has been carried out, there is still poor compliance with recommendations for sleep. Recently, the CDC released yet another information packet underscoring the need for sleep and how sleepy most of us are. It is a very real concern and one which requires attention but who's listening? Now, with the weight of the CDC behind it, it should receive more attention.

## Sleepy Nations

An astonishing 35% of Americans aren't getting enough sleep and when it comes to specific professions, they are getting a lot less than the recommended seven hours. In particular, those in medicine and other forms of shift workers are at great risk of sleepiness and prone to accidents.

Inspection of the 2014 US Census for workers over the age of 16 clearly shows that over six million workers are on their way to work between midnight and 5 AM. On the other end of the spectrum, close to 10 million workers begin the trip to work between 4 PM and midnight. How sleepy are many of them? Look around at the trains, buses and cars and you'll see a lot of yawning, coffee drinking or nodding off and you need no other information.

As *Wayne Giles, MD*, Director of CDC Division of Population Health, has said in a release from that government institution, *"as a nation we are not getting enough sleep. Lifestyle changes such as going to bed at the same time each night, rising at the same time each morning, and turning off or removing televisions, computers, or mobile devices from the bedroom, can help people get the healthy sleep they need."*

But are we doing as he suggests? Of course, we're not farmers anymore and our lives have changed drastically since the Industrial Revolution that took place at the turn of the 20th Century. Henry Ford's development of the assembly line in factories increased the temptations to stay up later and toss our sleep needs aside. Factories could, in fact, remain active for the entire day and night thanks to the light bulb.

It's hard to deny ourselves some modern-day pleasures, especially after a day of work where we have been left feeling we needed some form of relaxation and enjoyment. Sleep may not be on that agenda. Or we may believe we can catch up on lost sleep on the weekend. But can we?

Giles isn't alone in his stated concern that our society is making it harder and harder to get an adequate amount of sleep. One eminent sleep researcher, *Dr. Charles A. Czeisler*, Baldino Professor of Sleep Medicine at Harvard Medical School, has been quoted regarding how corporate America refuses to recognize the necessity of sleep and even lionizes those who sleep less.

As Giles said, *"We'd never say, 'That person is a great worker! He's drunk all the time!' Yet we continue to celebrate people who sacrifice sleep for work."* He was, of course, referring to the fact that lack of sleep is just as bad or even worse than being drunk no matter where you are or what you're doing. Working 100 hours a week is not a badge of honor. It is an indication of impending poor health.

Neither Giles nor Czeisler are alone in their considering sleep deprivation as something to be avoided and sleepy workers, as they well know, should not be viewed as super beings. The library of books and magazine articles on the topic of sleep deprivation grows daily despite the continued drumbeat of those who laud their ability to remain sleepless.

But we still hear the titans of industry and politics beating their chests on their own assumed merit of defeating sleep. Unfortunately, some see it as a sign of power. But it's not. The next time someone tells you how little sleep they require, you might consider that it's not all that good for them. Who are they fooling? When you try to function on less sleep, there is always a downside.

## Sleeplessness bragging and immorality

Sleep hasn't always been viewed as a vital necessity. Even men like the eminent Protestant minister, *Cotton Mather*, belittled those who would sleep. In one of his sermons he is said to have a decidedly negative opinion that any excess of sleep was sinful and, with true Puritan spirit, believed that those of his flocks who slept should be out working.

One wonders how *Cotton Mather* conceived what an actual "excess of sleep" would be? Just how many hours were righteous and how many more sinful according to his estimations? Mather didn't leave us any guidance on that one. Remember that he was also a vigorous supporter of the Salem witch trials and you have an idea of how wrathful he could be on any number of topics.

*Benjamin Franklin*, one of the Founding Fathers of the United States, inventor, ambassador and the man who organized the US postal service, was also fervently against sleep which he saw as better left to the grave where there would be plenty of time for it. I wonder how many hours of sleep he got each night and whether or not he napped during the day. We have no way of knowing, so his dismissal of sleep may have been totally personal.

Today, we know there is science behind our need for sleep and it is being tested and researched in Sleep Medicine. Where were we before Sleep Medicine was accepted and what did we believe? Despite the advent of this important medical specialty, there are still those who view sleep as an idol waste of valuable time.

Look what one executive had to say on the topic. He claimed he never sleeps more than 3 to 4 hours a night because he believes you can't be competitive in business if you sleep. It's a sentiment echoed by a number of other reasonably successful corporate executives.

*Marissa Mayer*, formerly of Yahoo, stated that she only sleeps 4 to 6 hours a night but takes a one week vacation every four months. The very talented and successful designer, apparel executive and movie director, *Tom Ford*, says he only needs three or four hours sleep a night.

The famous novel-writing *Brontë sisters* (Charlotte and Emily) were chronic insomniacs who, allegedly, walked around the dining room table until sleep overcame them. There may be some truth to that, but it may also be the pressures of their endeavors that caused the state of neglected sleep.

In addition to those I've mentioned so far, we can include *Margaret Thatcher*, former Prime Minister of Great Britain (who developed Alzheimer's), *Barack Obama*, and *Sir Isaac Newton* (who was said to sleep only two hours a night). Do great minds need less sleep? Not necessarily, but as in so many things, one size does not fit all. For some people they can sleep in brief snippets, while others require a full seven hours.

*Leonardo da Vinci*, supposedly slept two hours a night and, for the rest of the day and night got only 15-minute microsleep periods.

*Thomas Edison* groused about sleep as being for the lazy and claimed he only slept three hours a night but kept cots in all his laboratories so he could nap at many times during the day. Brain cleaning at work? Possibly.

## A sleep deprivation stunt

In 1959, New York City disk jockey Peter Tripp decided he would remain awake for 200 hours while he was on the air. It wasn't exactly just for publicity because money people contributed for the stunt was to go to The March of Dimes charity.

Sitting in a glass booth in Times Square, New York City, Tripp proceeded to begin a journey that would have an ending he never anticipated. During the show he did take stimulants to remain awake, however.

Medical personnel were monitoring him, and he seemed to do just fine as he went about his disk jockey chores. But after 100 hours of no sleep, he could no longer do simple math or recite the alphabet. When he reached 120 hours, he began to hallucinate, became paranoid and ran into the street when approached by one of the scientists.

Toward the end of the ordeal, which he did complete, he believed that he wasn't Peter Tripp but someone else. Seemingly, he was fine after 24 hours of sleep, but his life took several unpleasant turns after the stunt.

Tripp lost his job, was divorced by his wife and was then involved in the record company payola scandal of the 1990s that took a number of famous disk jockeys down with it and their careers were ruined.

# CHAPTER 7

# How much sleep do you need?

◆ ◆ ◆

*Though sleep is called our best friend,*
*it is a friend who often keeps us waiting! - Jules Verne*

Just how much sleep should you be getting on average each day? Usually, most people may say 6-7 hours is adequate and their view may be that 8 hours is just too much time to spend sleeping. Of course, in this rapidly-changing world we live in, more and more sleep has been seen as an indulgence rather than a necessity. It's similar with vacations, isn't it?

Some may boast about how little sleep they require, but this attitude, besides being decidedly unhealthy, is truly unwise now that you know a bit about sleep and what it does for us. Deny yourself sleep and pay the piper might be a good thing to keep in mind.

Experts in the field, such as those at the National Sleep Foundation (NSF), have provided us with a few guidelines and I've included some of their information here.

The NSF found that a greater amount of sleep is required from birth (anywhere from 14-17 hours of sleep) to just about the beginning of the teen years where we need, on average, 8-10 hours. Then the requirement for sleep pretty much stabilizes toward age 18 and may drop off a bit in older adults.

These are recommendations and may not be totally appropriate for everyone. It is necessary, therefore, that each individual monitor their sleep pattern to determine what works best for them.

No hard and fast rule here, just some averages and fluctuations within each age group are considered normal. It's hard to believe that just a decade ago a medical researcher actually said *there was no reason for anyone to sleep.* I wonder what he was thinking and what he believes today.

If we know that animals die if they are prevented from sleeping, what would that researcher think would happen to any of we mere mortals from a lack of sleep? Maybe he was just posing the question to arouse some interest in the whole subject of sleep and our requirements, so let's give him that bit of latitude.

## Sleep debt and its consequences/resolution

Now that you've had a chance to review the facts presented and to estimate where you may lie on this sleep continuum, how are you doing? Are you getting what is considered adequate for your age and activity group or not?

Very important question. It may mean you're headed for some problems in your everyday life as a consequence of what will be discussed in the next few paragraphs.

Consider this scenario. Suppose you have a job or some responsibility that keeps you from what is determined to be the optimum amount of sleep you should be getting. Well, there's a term for the result from that lack of sleep and it's called "sleep debt." This, as much as other debt, is truly disturbing because it may not be easily remedied.

As described by sleep experts, you calculate sleep debt simply by taking the number of hours you should be sleeping and subtracting the number of hours you are actually sleeping. The result is your debt and it can weigh quite heavily on you. No one wants to be in debt and this particular form of debt exacts a high price from you both physically and mentally.

Sleep debt is responsible for a lack of clarity in your thinking, vision problems, impaired driving, mood changes, anxiety and memory difficulties. Makes sense doesn't it that if you are sleep deprived you would not be functioning efficiently. Put it another way, if you wish, it would mean you're not running on all your mental and physical internal cylinders. Sort of like a car that has one poorly functioning cylinder. It makes a clanging noise, doesn't it? But that clang warns you to get to the mechanic. In this instance, YOU are your own mechanic since you should be able to control your sleep needs.

How will you be sensitive to the warning signs of sleep deprivation, especially if you like to think you can always function on less sleep than other people? Really not something to crow about because you may be getting deeper into debt than you realized. Then, too, this debt will be hard to erase or may not be able to be removed.

Can you store up hours of sleep and make a withdrawal during those times when work or other activities permit you to sleep? Probably not.

As our cultures have quickly implemented the 24-hour workday, 7-days-a-week style of business, the question of sleep has risen to a point of contention. If someone wants to get ahead in the digital world, they are derided for wanting a normal sleep routine and some type of normal life.

The only path to the top of Silicon Valley appears to be the one which the original titans charted. That trek meant sleeping in the office, under a desk or slumped over a table. Ever read what both *Steve Jobs* and *Bill Gates* did on many nights?

Jobs slept in his office, when he slept, much of the time. The music genius *Prince* worked all hours of the day and night and didn't have a bedroom in his home.

None of those sleep situations are acceptable but the matter has been viewed as a joke of sorts as one online business blog saw it. *Elan Musk* freely admits that he has slept in his Tesla car factory for weeks on end until the production run was over.

A symbol of the new elite has been the erstwhile hoodie of *Marc Zuckerberg* of Facebook fame. Zuckerberg, as you may know, has pulled all-nighter coding sessions. It is still seen as a form of torturous creativity and recreation at the same time for coders to engage, just for fun, in coding for 24-hours at a time. Usually, they are in competition with each other to complete some creative task.

One recent online article took sleeping on the job all in fun and offered a number of rather creative but totally unrealistic scenarios. How can you get the sleep you need or at least nap a bit to help you drag your weary body through the seemingly endless day, they asked?

How about sneaking into the restroom and nodding out in a stall, going off to a conference room without a glass wall and getting a few winks or even faking it big time by wearing a hoodie (big with the under-30 crowd) and sunglasses while sitting at your computer?

Some people do try to sleep under their desks, and I have heard of a young man doing that. Of course, the entire article was all in fun but there's a very big dollop of truth there. Everyone is craving sleep, but no one can admit it or even manage to get the sleep they need. The business world just doesn't look kindly on sleeping.

Did you know that online instructors at universities are told they are to be available to their students (who are all around the world) 24/7 and must respond to email within 1-4 hours after its receipt? How can anyone do a job with that expectation? They, therefore, usually work a 16-hour day (at a computer) with email and reading papers from students and it's a seven-days-a week schedule.

I'd call that a grinding one and I can't imagine that many last very long at it. You may think working at home is a dream job, but not at this pace. A question that comes to mind is how does it affect the work product of students who are taking those courses. How might it affect grades if an instructor wants to get done and hand out grades which weren't earned?

In his book, "*Dangerously Sleepy: Overworked Americans and the Cult of Manly Wakefulness*," Alan Derickson noted that men had learned to see sleep not only as an indication of laziness, but a state to be avoided. It is masculinity at its most dangerous in terms of health and safety. Who pays the price? All of us.

Derickson also stated that, "*as methods of production became more capital-intensive, it became an imperative to make sure that equipment did not sit idle... There were industries – paper and steel – that couldn't shut down and needed people around the clock to run and maintain that equipment.*"

Part of this current belief in the disdain for sleep was fostered by

*Thomas Edison* whose estimate of how long he slept each day may have been what has been found in sleep experiments. One finding was that everyone seems to have a poor ability to say how much sleep they actually get. In addition, they can't accurately evaluate how competent they are to function on that amount of sleep. We're biased to think well of ourselves and some engage in more of this than others.

One of Edison's inventions, the lightbulb, would earn him the moniker of "Father of the Night Shift." How many people didn't think so kindly of this "modern invention" intruding into their lives? I'll bet a lot of people and many of them discovered that the night shift was an unexpected difficulty.

## Sleeplessness is not a badge of honor

One of the unfortunate aspects of our wonderful digital media is that anyone who is a successful entrepreneur will have access to an excessive amount of time either on TV or the Internet where they extol the value of not sleeping. We still hear, unfortunately as I've said, about media or computer moguls spending unreasonable hours of time working on programming. Corporate leaders tell us that all you need is three hours sleep a night. It's all in some distorted belief that Mother Nature can be fooled and they know her game and how to play it better than she.

A quick scan of the obituaries in major newspapers reveals how much the titans of industry gave for their corporate gains as we see men and even women in their 50s and 60s dying suddenly. Look at their photos and you may experience a sense of disbelief that they weren't 20 years older than their actual age. Sleep loss takes its toll if we fail to pay attention to it.

Almost weekly we read about the deaths of company men in various parts of the world, like Japan, who died from overwork. There are articles about young interns in financial institutions, too, who pull extraordinarily long workdays in hopes of being offered jobs that promise a super salary and prestige.

TV shows provide a vivid image of young attorneys who want to make partner but have to fill client log hours that are beyond unbelievable. One executive I knew called it "smoke-and-mirrors" time because he knew he couldn't manage the hours but they had to be calculated. Yes, he lied on his and everyone else's log sheets.

With the advent of the light bulb, the factories could remain continuously producing and the labor force would be required to bend to new shifts that could prove to be detrimental to their health and safety. It wasn't just health and safety at risk. Family life was disrupted.

It's not that the brain is lazy, but one immediate fact that becomes obvious was that shifts were related to an increase in accidents with the revised shifts. Sleepy workers have problems around any complex machinery.

Current research is pointing to things we would never suspect might interfere with our sleep. Do you take a cell phone or iPad or any other electronic device to bed with you at night? Even the glow of these devices can disrupt your best efforts to sleep, so it's in your best interest to do a quick scan of your devices now. If you need your cell phone near your bed, turn it over so the light won't show.

Innocent though these items may seem, their glow has the ability to spark activity in your eyes, which then gets translated by your brain into a distorted sleep-wake cycle. This seemingly innocuous message actually disrupts your body's ability to remain in a state that signals it's time to go to sleep.

Take a look at these tips passed along to us from many of the sleep experts in the field and see which ones are most agreeable to you and which will work for you.

**PRINT THIS OUT** and put it on the fridge or someplace where you'll see it frequently as a reminder to you:

*Go to sleep when you're sleepy or if you're in bed and not sleepy, try reading a book for a bit.*

Twenty minutes and not asleep yet? Get up and do something in another room until you feel sleepy. May not always be possible but give it a try.

What helps you to relax before you go to bed? Warm bath or shower, light snack or a bit of reading?

Awaken at the same time each morning, go to bed at the same time. Schedules can be a big help.

Try to keep everything on a regular basis. Might seem a bit obsessive, but it works.

Bed is for sleeping. It's not for TV, eating meals or talking on the phone. I don't care what Hugh Hefner of Playboy did, it won't work for you.

No rigorous exercise before you go to bed to go to sleep. It just energizes you and that defeats the whole purpose here.

Tell yourself that this is time to sleep, not worry about the day or tomorrow.

Make sure the room is dark and quiet and remember that cool is better for a bedroom. Suggestions for room temperature are around 65 degrees F.

Another tip might be to try one of those lights that awaken you by slowly emulating the sun coming up and brighten in the morning to bring you just enough light to wake you up. It's pleasant.

## Sleep debt, kids and ADHD

Children are especially vulnerable since many of them use their devices in their beds before they go to sleep (Kleeman, 2017). The result is that they have sleep disruptions that can cause problems during their waking hours such as paying attention, remaining alert or applying themselves to learning. They are, in fact, accumulating that sleep debt I just talked about, but no one in the home may be aware of this or may fail to see it as a serious issue.

A grouchy kid may just be a sleepy kid and not a child with behavioral problems that can best be fixed with more sleep. Too often these children may be misdiagnosed as having behavioral/mental health problems and requiring powerful medications to address a non-existent attention deficit hyperactivity disorder (ADHD). For further information you might do a search to see what the eminent psychiatrist Dr. Allen Frances has to say about children, ADHD and medications.

Sleep and how it relates to children reaching their full potential is also a concern in other parts of the world. A study (Dawson, 2016) of 1,000 children in Great Britain showed that sleep was being sacrificed, especially around exam time.

Student results broke out in the following manner:

83% of teens admit their sleep is affected by stress and worry
56% admit to regularly cramming all their studying for an exam into
    one night
82% used their bed for studying
26% of teens drink energy/caffeine drinks to stay awake even though
    we know that's not prudent
46% find themselves snacking more often

When questioned about their children's sleep habits, 80% of the parents believed there was no problem. Yet, over 30% of the pupils were referred for
mental health or sleep problems and one of the most frequent complaints
they had, in addition to lack of sleep, was anxiety.

For many students, even though they went to bed at 10PM, they didn't
get to sleep until the early hours of the morning. Some children reported
they got only an average of 2-1/2 hours sleep during exam time.

Another study of over 2,000 school children found that just over 35%
of teens reported that they watched TV to help them go to sleep, almost
15% of girls studied used computer games in bed and 60% used music as
a sleep aid.

Half of the kids read books to fall asleep and the researchers found that,
with the exception of books, the use of other forms of media meant these
teens got fewer hours of sleep. As a result, these kids were significantly
more tired than others who used books. So, the answer for parents concerned about sleepy kids? Give them books to read in bed before they go to
sleep. No TV or computers.

One additional note may be useful here. Reading or studying something and then going to sleep actually is a great aid in consolidating information and facilitates learning any material. So, read something you want
to learn just before you go to sleep, and you will have an additional benefit.

Sleep and the lack of it is now being considered, as Dr. Allen Frances
believes, as a major contributory factor in Attention Deficit Hyperactivity
Disorder (ADHD) where children are unable to concentrate and are in

motion constantly. It is a behavioral disorder, but it may also be related to the hormonal changes that come with sleep deprivation.

The explosion of this diagnosis has led some mental health professionals to question the diagnosis. The activity is a question now of whether these kids are truly being adequately evaluated and medicated for a disorder that may not be psychiatric in nature at all. How often do parents know how much sleep their kids are getting?

Look at the British study where fully 80% of parents were totally unaware their kids weren't getting enough sleep. How was that possible?

Writing in Psychiatric Times, *Drs. James Dillon* and *Ronald Chervin* noted that prior research had shown that "*very modest changes in sleep duration can substantially affect the neurobehavioral function of children.*" The research they cite seems to indicate that an underlying psychiatric disorder is leading to sleep disturbances. However, the question can be rephrased to ask whether the sleep disorder is manifesting in a behavioral disorder in the daytime and being misperceived as a psychiatric disorder.

Then, too, we must remember the high incidence of utilization of digital media in the form of smart phones, iPads, computers and TVs with their blue-light element in the mix. Apple noted the problem with the blue light from iPhones and issued a fix for it. The situation, therefore, is not necessarily one of an underlying psychiatric disorder and all factors must be added in before we can come to any meaningful conclusion.

Rather than medicating a child initially for a behavioral daytime disorder, perhaps consideration should be given to limiting the use of digital media by these children. Keeping sleep logs regarding this restriction and their daytime behavior would be helpful. Note the hours of sleep they get each evening and the quality of their sleep.

This would only seem reasonable since the number of children being placed on psychoactive medication is disturbingly high. You may wish to review the CDC report and statistical maps on the distribution of ADHD diagnosis in the country which were published on their website on January 4, 2016.

In 2016, 6.1 million US children between the ages of 2 through17 were diagnosed with ADHD and ages 2 though 5 *"increased by more than 50% from the 2007-2008 survey to the 2011-12 survey."* There has been a dramatic increase but why? Is sleep an unknown factor here?

The matter of sleep and all types of psychiatric disorders requires a careful consideration of ALL factors before any determination can be made. Doing otherwise is unethical and potentially harmful.

## Light and your sleep

Little did we know that tiny light receptors in our eyes, probably related to the same mechanism which tells birds it's time to migrate, have an incredible influence and power over our wakefulness. Small lights which may seem to us to be too insignificant to be noticed are picked up by these alert cells. The cells are constantly scanning for any signal to them to reset our internal (or circadian) clocks. A resetting is not what we want done because it interferes with all bodily functioning.

Evolutionarily coded to respond in a protective way to light, the cells continue to perform the actions for which they were first produced in our ancestors. At this point in time, we no longer need to consider migrating with herds or relative to the weather. But these little cells keep on working away to keep that clock performing as it did millions of years ago.

What are those little light receptor cells doing? Feverishly, they are promoting or inhibiting the production of a vital sleep-related hormone, melatonin. As one Harvard sleep researcher, *Stephen Lockley*, indicated in a published interview, even dim light can interfere with a person's melatonin secretion.

This body clock is located in a small structure in the brain known as the suprachiasmatic nucleus close to the connecting point for your optic nerve for your eyes (the optic chiasma). Birds have this structure just behind a thin boney plate in the front of their heads.

Light striking this area sets off a chemical reaction that tells the birds when it's time to hit the road and go wherever their group does for the winter or spring. Our brains have this structure even though we don't engage in migratory behavior, except in the case of North Americans who flee south in the winter to escape the cold and are, therefore, dubbed "snow birds."

## Sleeping medications

Sleeping pills have an interesting history but, some of it is shocking and regrettable. During the 1920s or 30s there was little regulation over many addictive medications and some were sold over-the-counter. Today, these addictive medications can present problems when casually dismissed as nothing more than a sleep aid. One illustration we can use is the problems surrounding the distribution of one of the premier sleeping medications, Ambien.

Halcion was previously the darling of the benzodiazepines because it produced rapid onset of sleep and appeared to have exactly what persons who had insomnia were seeking; restful sleep. The problems with Halcion were recognized once persons who used it indicated that they were having serious next-day memory loss and increasing depression.

In Britain, it reached a point where up to 800,000 people were using it and 7 million patients were using it in the United States. European authorities withdrew the medication and other countries limited the dosages available after reports of disconcerting side effects.

Sleep medications are generally seen as a treatment of last resort, especially if they are be used on a chronic basis. The many reasons for not taking a sleep medication nightly can be outlined succinctly in one word, side effects. The side effects of sleep medications, which may not have clearly been outlined sufficiently for consumers, are troubling and need to be considered whenever a sleep medication is prescribed.

Medications, any medication for whatever illness or disorder you may have, come with side effects. Side effects may be slight, common, or rare and some of them can be quite disturbing.

Singling out any one medication is especially onerous and not appropriate because many of the medications are helpful for scores of people. Some individuals may experience problems, where others have no problems whatsoever, so it really is an individual case of your body's ability to tolerate a specific medication. Not everyone will be able to tolerate the same medication that their friends or family or associates can and that's normal. Normal is a range from no side effects to severe side effects and everywhere in between. The determination must be made, individually, by you and your physician who is prescribing for you.

Occasionally, a medication, even a sleep medication, may originally present problems but after what is known as a "challenge," the medication may not affect the person as before. Therefore, it is often the case that a medication that once couldn't be taken, can be taken at some future date. Keep that in mind because it may prove to be helpful to you.

Doing an Internet search, you can easily find that of the millions of people who have taken medications, some have had very serious and bizarre side effects. Unfortunately, Ambien has been involved in several high-profile cases.

One case, in 2009, involved a man who had taken Ambien and then killed eight people. Another case involved a man who was driving and collided with a number of cars. He had no recall. The singer, Eminem, has stated that, as a result of taking Ambien he had lost five years of his memory and the actor John Stamos indicated that he had become addicted to the medication.

I should point out that addiction to medication simply means that he could not get to sleep at night without taking the medication. Often, however, there may be a contrary effect (aka paradoxical effect) and the medication itself, not specifically Ambien, may cause insomnia rather than helping a person get to sleep. Even former-Representative Patrick Kennedy, who as a member of Congress, was involved in a car accident after taking this medication. Several famous film stars have indicated serious side effects that caused them to engage in bizarre behavior. One indicated he almost drove his car over a cliff while on Ambien. Yes, these cases make the headlines, but they do not make the case for the medication being totally inappropriate for many people.

## Autism and melatonin

Children with autism, according to a recent study of over 125 children in 24 sites both in the United States and the European Union, were given melatonin, the naturally-occurring hormone that helps us sleep. The results, while still requiring further evaluation, seem to indicate that these children had significantly improved sleep from baseline, slept longer, fell asleep faster and had longer uninterrupted sleep as compared to their normal, regular sleep activity.

Parents also indicated that there appeared to be some positive behavioral changes which were beneficial in terms of aggression and their ability to maintain their activity level, i.e., less hyperactivity.

Although promising, the researchers did indicate that there are potential problems associated with long-term use of melatonin and they are not indicating that it should be considered without more extensive testing.

# CHAPTER 8

# Sleep's Many Features

◆ ◆ ◆

*The world of men is dreaming, it has gone mad in its sleep,*
*and a snake is strangling it, but it can't wake up. - D. H. Lawrence*

Studying human sleep and the disorders identified so far may have opened: new avenues to understanding what motivates us to sleep and why we need it, but it also points to how similar we may be to animals. Animals? Yes, animals and how some portions of our brain may function in ways which evolution plotted as a means of survival. In fact, we may be more similar to animals than we think.

## Seabirds, wild animals and sleep

We know what causes birds to migrate as a function of the light in the area where they currently reside, but how do birds sleep and how much sleep do they need? Might we learn something about our sleep activities from a study of bird sleep? Perhaps we can learn from birds after all.

We might assume that, based on the size of their brains and the need for clearing, birds need a lot of sleep. Not so easy to know, however. It's pretty difficult to study the sleep habits of wild birds and the brain activity that stimulates it. But it seems they sleep very little, or they sleep in a different manner than we do. But their brains and our's do share something in common.

An interesting thing about birds is how they sleep and it's pretty startling. It may also tell us something about our own sleep patterns and disturbances of sleep, such as sleepwalking.

Did you know that some bird species (Rattenborg, 2016), such as frigate birds that fly over the open oceans, sleep in flight for journeys that can last up to 10 days? The trick here is that evolution allows the two hemispheres of their brains to work independently (one awake while the other is asleep) or both can shut down together.

Unbelievable I think, but frigate birds aren't unique. Similar findings have turned up in swifts, sandpipers, some song birds and other seabirds and wild animals.

Brain sections of what is known as our "primitive" brain (the limbic system) take over our alertness-while-asleep function. It's a similar one found in wild animals that can spring to action while asleep and avoid becoming dinner.

For animals, this primitive mechanism is truly vital as it may be, in some cases, for us. We react much more to light in terms of sleep/wake cycles, but we still use that hemispheric divide; one side being "asleep" while the other side of our brain watches over us and our brain turns on the watchman. Have you ever given any thought to that? I don't think any of us have because it's an astounding discovery. How could we still be somehow "awake" to scout our environment for potential danger as we sleep?

## The primitive brain and sleep

How might the sleep habits of seabirds or wild animals (that do the uni-hemisphere shuffle while asleep) tell us something about human sleep? Studies, in fact, have found that we have areas of our brain that are vigilant even while we sleep. A similar activity occurs while we are under general anesthesia; we still hear what's going on in the environment and can be affected by it. These areas make decisions, without our prompting, to remain asleep or wake up in response to something disturbing.

This is especially true when we move to a new environment (Tamaki et al., 2016) where it is highly important to monitor our surroundings for any sign of danger. It is known as the First Night Effect (FNE) and anyone who's ever moved has probably experienced it and noted every little creak and noise in the night. For some it will be a sleepless night for that first night or even a few afterward.

Our brain enters default mode as we doze off and those primitive areas act as the night watchman that goes to work without any encouragement. Ever notice how a change in where you live may lead to that first night not being one of restful sleep? How often must people traveling on business trips contend with this sleepless night effect as they go from hotel to hotel in different cities?

## DSPS or ASPS? What does it mean?

DSPS (Delayed Sleep Phase Syndrome) boils down to when you fall asleep as well as when you wake up, preferably, as well as questions of lifestyle and aging. Come to think of it, these two disorders may not really be disorders. What may be happening is more a question of activity level and involvement in various efforts in our lives and even retirement. Allow me to explain.

DSPS is of unknown cause and is an irregularity in the circadian (sleep) rhythms which are controlled by that internal biological clock that sets our sleep-wake patterns. Some people who experience this type of disorder are those who have had head injuries or serious illness but there is another group, too; teenagers and college students. These students have had neither injury nor illness but experience this sleep-wake disruption. Explore that a bit and you will understand why there would seem to be some who might have more control over it.

Teenagers and college students, generally, have one thing in common and that is that they tend to go to sleep later at night when they are doing their homework or engaging in social activities. This means that they may not get to sleep until 3 AM in the morning and, naturally, experience great difficulty getting up and remaining alert during the day. Originally seen as a sleep disorder, the degree and episodic nature of DSPS may, in fact, lead to some confusion. The question, of course, is whether or not it should be considered a true sleep disorder.

Anyone leading a DSPS life is at risk for academic difficulties or even problems in retaining information or being active on a job-site. Students, in particular, have been shown to utilize shortened sleep at night and come home after school for a much-needed nap. Only much later in the day do they "pick up speed" and begin to function optimally. In fact, some experts have noted that these individuals seem to function best after midnight. I suppose you could call them "night owls."

Two thoughts that have been offered as elements contributing to the development or the continuance of this disorder are both electric lighting (of course computer screens must be added here too) and our culture which is a go-go society.

The thinking is that, if you are not active and doing things, there must be something wrong. Succumbing to this way of thinking results in a whole host of problems for the individual centered around sleep or the lack of it.

Advanced Sleep Phase Syndrome (ASPS), on the other hand is something that is experienced usually by persons who may be elderly, retired or have a low tolerance for stress. They become quite sleepy during the early evening and generally would go to bed between 8 and 9 PM. It may be perfectly fine to go to sleep early, but these individuals find it difficult to sleep throughout the night. So, they find themselves getting up at one or two in the morning when they would prefer to sleep until 6 or 7 AM.

What do you do when you wake up at 3 AM and you can't seem to go back to sleep? We've offered some suggestions later in this book and one I might offer here is for you to engage in some minimally active task such as reading a book. Do NOT watch TV or use a computer, unless the screens have a means of filtering out the blue light which they emit. You'll understand that later.

Again, this may be more a matter of lifestyle and lack of stimulation in life rather than a circadian rhythm problem. Our cultures generally value working and maintaining an active involvement in some creative effort on an ongoing basis. We know this from social interactions. What is the first question anyone may ask you when you are in a new setting and they have just met you?

Yes, of course, it's, "What do you do?" You immediately understand that what you are being asked is *what type of work you do*. It can be disconcerting, upsetting or energizing. If you are not working, what sort of answer do you give which will permit you to maintain your self-esteem and still seem like a worthwhile person?

Of course, there are genetic inheritance factors involved in all of our biological functioning and it may be here, too. I once worked with a man who was married and had three preteen children.

For that family, it was quite normal for them to go grocery shopping at 10 PM at night. You might find this shocking, but for them it was absolutely normal. I have no idea how the kids got up in the morning, but he never showed any sleepiness at work during the day where he produced as expected as a salesman who was highly valued.

## How much light is disturbing?

In terms of light, a mere eight lux—a level of brightness exceeded by most table lamps and about twice that of a night light—has an effect on our sleep. It's yet another hormonal effect of which we may not be aware. And it's not only the light, but the actual color of the light which can have a powerful effect on the production of melatonin, the sleep hormone.

Blue light is the most forceful suppressor of melatonin and what is the color most associated with night lights, computer screens, iPads and cell phones? You guessed it, it's blue light of course. LED and compact fluorescent bulbs are among the worst offenders, too. In fact, blue light was twice as potent at holding that wonderful sleep-promoting melatonin at bay as any other colors.

What to do? A somewhat unusual idea was to switch your night lights to red from the usual bulb in these units. Of course, this may take some adjustment on your part and cause a few unusual questions to be directed your way, but you have research to back you up on this, so do it.

Some people try wearing blue light-blocking sunglasses in bed as they use their digital toys. But you've already heard that your bed shouldn't be a place to work and yet people do it. Again, sunglasses may not be something for everyone but it does block out the blue light that's going to disrupt your sleep cycle. You can also buy a filter to place over your computer screen to inhibit the blue light from coming through. The computer will work fine and you'll be able to use it. Question yourself, however, about the reason you're using your computer or other items in bed and not using it strictly for sleep.

The eyes are the portal of entry for any light. Even if your eyes are closed, it may still be possible for light signals to get through your thin eyelids.

Why do you suppose some people find it impossible to sleep without a sleep mask? Some may be even more susceptible to the "call of the wild" of these receptors and additional attempts must be employed to block out the offending light. No doubt that there are areas of our brain still vigilant as we try to sleep.

## Far from the urban lights

Most of us, live in an urban environment where there is plenty of light not only in our homes from our many devices, but from the outside in terms of streetlights and local buildings or businesses. We may assume, therefore, that because we are "urban villagers" we are subject to an unnatural sleep environment. What about a different environment that didn't have all this light in it? That assumption was put to the test in a remote village in Madagascar

The villagers who have neither electricity nor artificial light in the area, we would assume, would benefit from living in a more natural environment devoid of all of these sleep-disturbances contraptions of modern life. We now know that isn't the case because even in areas of the world where there isn't the incessant glow of streetlights there is a disruption of sleep. No such luck.

The researchers studying their sleep habits came to a somewhat shocking conclusion when they looked at their data. The villagers actually had shorter, poorer sleep than people in the U.S. Why might that be?

Even though the villagers maintained a regular daytime-to-sleep time schedule, going to sleep around 7:30PM, they awakened at 5:30AM, or an hour before sunrise in their area.

Nighttime sleep was often disrupted by sounds in the environment, local dogs, sounds on tin roofs or loud neighbors. Often, once awakened during the night, they would not go immediately back to bed to sleep but might remain awake for a time and then return to sleep.

What is different here since the villagers didn't report being sleepy during the day and didn't complained about their lack of sleep? They nap during the day for up to one hour. The study provoked such interest in the researchers that they intend to carry it out around the world to tap into the sleep habits of various cultures.

Natural sleep is wonderful and necessary, but not everyone gets to enjoy it. Sleep researchers, so far, have differentiated the categories of disorders related to sleep.

## The major categories of sleep disorders are:

Insomnias
Sleep-related breathing disorders
Hypersomnias of central origin
Circadian rhythm sleep disorders
Parasomnias
Sleep-related movement disorders
Isolated symptoms, apparently normal variants and unresolved issues
Other sleep disorders

Detailed explanations of each category and the disorders subsumed in each category may be obtained by referring to the "*International Classification of Sleep Disorders*" published by The American Academy of Sleep Medicine. It can usually be found in the reference section of larger libraries.

The purpose of my book isn't to be a quasi-textbook on sleep, but an informative primer of sorts intended to explain sleep and to offer assistance to anyone experiencing sleep disruptions that may be self-remediated. Another purpose is to make a case for the necessity of sleep as it relates to our lives, whether at work, at school or at home.

As I've always told my college and graduate students, I am opening a door and it is your choice to go through the doorway to learn or not to learn. You decide because I've shown you the door and I've opened it just a tiny bit for a peek inside. Now it's up to you to initiate a journey or not.

## Sleep and the adolescent brain

An additional point that must be made here regarding sleep and brain volume relates to academic performance in children. Researchers were, admittedly, shocked to discover that sleep, with regard to bedtime during the week and on weekends, had a high correlation with adolescent brain volume in specific brain regions.

The result of this decrease in sleep was, again, directly related to academic performance in children who were getting inadequate sleep. Remember, the brain is developing until between 21-25 years of age, according to latest estimates, and during this time there is major brain structural change taking place.

Everyone sees the growth spurt in children but there's another growth spurt they didn't understand. Consider this brain "growth spurt" and sleep bedtime assumes a new role in actual physical changes in structures of the adolescent brain. A brain in an adolescent deprived of adequate sleep may turn out to be a brain stymied in growth of vital structures indispensable for performing well in school and life.

Researchers hadn't expected what they found and cautioned against hasty conclusions but suggest it might be an area to consider in any academic plans for adolescents who were not performing well in school. So, if there's an adolescent in your home, consider their sleep time and, possibly, keeping a sleep journal and matching it with their school performance.

## Sleep in children with autism

Sleep disorders may be more common in children with autism spectrum disorders (ASD) and researchers have estimated that the incidence of a sleep disorder may be anywhere up to 80% of children with this diagnosis. The most common problems that these children experience is difficulty falling asleep, inconsistent sleep routines, restlessness or poor sleep quality and waking early and waking frequently.

Of course, lacking a good night's sleep affects the child's behavior and is disruptive to the entire family. At this point, researchers have not definitively identified the reason why these children have sleep problems, but they have several theories that they are looking into.

One theory is that there are some social cues involved in knowing when it's time to go to sleep at night. Also, even though a child with this disorder may see other children going to bed, they don't see that that is something they should be doing, too.

A second theory, which they are investigating, involves the normal sleep-related hormone, melatonin, which regulates our sleep-wake cycles. Children with ASD have been found to have both higher or lower levels of this hormone and therefore they have different responses during the night and the day. Such a release discrepancy from the usual discharge of this hormone would result in an inactivation of its ability to promote sleep when it's dark and wakeful activity during light hours. In fact, in some children, the exact reverse of the normal expression of melatonin occurs; high during the daytime and low at night.

The third theory that is being delved into is that children who have ASD are more sensitive to external stimuli and therefore are troubled by this when they are attempting to sleep. Even a simple opening of a door or movement of a blanket may result in an unexpected sleep disruption resulting in difficulty to return to restful sleep.

We also know that children with this syndrome have high levels of anxiety and therefore they are, once again, more likely to have a heightened startle response to any change in stimulation in the environment.

What are some of the resulting behavioral manifestations of sleep disorder in children with ASD? Researchers have found that they include aggression, depression, hyperactivity, irritability, increased behavioral problems, and problems in learning and performing cognitive tests. Of course, if a child cannot concentrate and is anxious, it is understood that will interfere with their ability to maintain concentration needed for attention to lessons and, therefore, to learn and to retain what they have learned.

CHAPTER 9

# Details of Sleep Disorders

◆ ◆ ◆

*Space and light and order. Those are the things that men need
just as much as they need bread or a place to sleep. Le Corbusier*

Sleep disorders fall primarily within one specific set of disorders known as the parasomnias which occur both in REM as well as NREM sleep. In other words, these disruptive sleep disorders can occur while we are dreaming in rapid eye movement (REM) or non-rapid eye movement (NREM) sleep. The hallmark of these disorders is the person engages in undesirable physical or verbal behaviors which may be noted by their bed partner or those in the area around them.

During these sleep-disruptive periods, the individual will have no awareness that they are performing certain actions or saying things. Once they return to sleep and awaken the next morning, they have amnesia for any of the events. The types of disorders which fall into the parasomnias include:

## *NREM group*

***Somnambulism:*** *sleepwalking most usual in children and often runs in families so relatives may have this problem, too.*

***Sleep terrors:*** *often associated with loud screams, signs of panic and possible harm to others or furniture. There is amnesia on the part of the individual once they awaken.*

*Bruxism (teeth grinding): usually associated with stress and anxiety*

*Restless legs syndrome: an inability to find a restful position for the legs while in bed and attempting to sleep. The result is non-restful sleep because of all the tossing and turning the individual engages in while in bed.*

## REM group

**RBD** (aka REM sleep behavior disorder), is a sleep state in which muscle activity is not restrained as it normally would be during sleep. The person, in response to highly disturbing dreams, attempts to respond to dream situations, resulting in potential injury to themselves or others. Bed partners may be injured during these episodes.

Again, there appears to be a relationship to gender and age with the greatest number of persons being male and over the age of 50. The disorder may be a reaction to some medications, including antidepressants.

**Recurrent sleep paralysis** where the individual cannot move upon awakening or when drifting off to sleep. Have you ever awakened during the night or early in the morning and found that you couldn't move? You felt able to think, but your body just wouldn't respond to your wishes and you were paralyzed. It is a disturbing feeling and can cause feelings of panic in anyone who experiences it, but it's not uncommon and, in fact, it's a part of natural sleep.

The paralysis can last from seconds to a few minutes and it is something that may come and go, happen once or twice a month and, for some people, not at all. No matter how many times it happens, it's not something you want to go through because you can neither move nor speak.

As one woman described it, when she was a teen, it was a regular part of her sleep and it did stop suddenly as she entered adulthood. But the feeling of paralysis was totally frightening and accompanied by a ringing in her ears.

The sensation came on at bedtime, during the night or upon awakening in the morning and she was afraid to tell anyone. She only began to realize she wasn't having a mental breakdown when she heard a co-worker discussing it during a coffee break.

The one thing that has been found to stand out about anyone who experiences regular sleep paralysis is that it's in persons who are sleep deprived. But it can also be related to the brain's ability to quiet muscle activity in order to promote continued sleep. We know that the major muscles of the body will experience this type of "paralysis" normally, so it would seem that some sleepers are waking up before their brains have shut off that sleep-related mechanism.

**Nightmares** which are truly terrifying dreams that arouse fear, terror and high anxiety in the sleeping person. At these times, the heart may race and the breathing may become increased as it would be in a person attempting to escape from something frightening.

I've provided a few of the more common sleep disorders here with a brief description of their characteristics. They are placed in no specific order, so please don't conclude that because sleep apnea is first that it is either the most common (although it is quite common) or the most serious. A complete listing of the currently accepted sleep disorders may be found in **International Classification of Sleep Disorders – Third Edition (ICSD-3) (Online).**

Remember something else, too. Sleep disorders may very well be much like other physical disorders in that they may not be clear-cut disorders but may have characteristics of several disorders.

First, however, give yourself an opportunity to gauge your sleepiness by using a favorite scale that's widely used, the Epworth Sleepiness Scale and be sure to complete the two scales we have at the end of the book in *Appendices B and C.*

## Epworth Sleepiness Scale

The Epworth Sleepiness Scale is widely used in the field of sleep medicine as a subjective measure of sleepiness. The scale is a list of eight situations in which you rate your tendency to become sleepy on a score of 0, no chance of dozing off to sleep, to 3, high chance of dozing. When you finish the test, add up the values of your responses. Your total score is based on a scale of 0 to 24.

The scale provides a rough estimate regarding possible excessive sleepiness that may require medical attention. Since it is a self-evaluation, it is *not a substitution for a professional evaluation* because any instrument that is totally dependent on a person's own perception of something has a high degree of uncertainty regarding whether it is a valid measure or not.

We have not reproduced the scale here. If you wish to see the actual scale, you can go to this link: *https://web.stanford.edu/~dement/epworth.html* at Stanford University in California, USA that will actually allow you to take a short form of the test and get your score. A lengthier scale is used by clinicians and that's the reason your score may not have the additional refinements that are found in the professional version.

Why didn't we provide the actual scale here? First, it is copyrighted and second, it would be unethical for me to do so. Scales such as this require that they be protected in order to ensure the results are as accurate as possible. If we were to publish them, as some unethical persons might, we would be doing a disservice to anyone who needed an evaluation and we would, in effect, be providing practice for anyone who wanted to cheat on the test.

Why not keep a record of when you feel you could nod off to sleep during the day, under what conditions and what you were doing at the time, as well as the environment? Also, keep a log of when you went to sleep the night before and how many hours of sleep you got. Call it a daily wakefulness diary, if you like and be sure to check it after at least one week to see if you can spot a trend.

It might be quite surprising when you do complete the scale. Also, be sure to drop to the end of this book for a link to a website which provides a scale to see if you're a "lark" or an "owl" in terms of sleep behavior.

We have provided a scale (*Appendix B*) at the end of this book, *The Morningness-Eveningness Scale*, which will help you to determine at which times of the day you do best. It's self-scored and provides guidance but *not a clinical impression*. For anything clinical, you should consult a sleep medicine specialist. Yes, you can think of it as also being a way of determining your "lark" or "owl" status.

## Sleep Apnea

Sleep apnea, also known as Obstructive Sleep Apnea (OSA), has become one of the more common sleep disorders found both in men and women as well as some children. It is characterized by frequent nighttime awakenings, without awareness, which results in excessive daytime sleepiness.

There is a specific cycle associated with sleep apnea and one of the hallmarks is snoring. So, anyone who is snoring loudly all of the time may be a candidate for a professional evaluation.

### *Sleep apnea cycle*

The cycle begins with a breathing pause after the initiation of sleep and it is associated with that snoring I mentioned. During this time, the throat airway proceeds to narrow and there is increased effort to breathe in. Once this begins, the brain, in effect, signals a period of oxygen starvation and the person awakens suddenly with a choking sensation. The entire cycle is triggered by that low blood oxygen level that has set off the brain's alarm system which is a monitor for inadequate oxygen.

The interrupted breathing may happen up to 500 times a night, resulting in poor sleep quality and lack of any awareness on the part of the individual that this has happened. All the person knows is that they never seem able to get a good, restful night's sleep. It's not until they are evaluated in a sleep lab that the disorder can correctly be diagnosed, and steps taken to utilize one of the many forms of treatment.

According to The National Sleep Foundation, over 18 million American adults have this sleep disorder. In children, the number with the disorder may be as high as 20% of those who snore habitually. Actual statistics regarding children may be difficult to gather, however, because of differences in monitoring children.

The causes of sleep apnea are varied and include:

Small upper airway (which includes a large tongue, tonsils or uvula)
Overweight individuals
Recessed chin, small jaw or large overbite

Large neck (in men that can be 17 in. or greater and in women 16 in.
 or greater)
Use of smoking products and alcohol
Age over 40
Ethnic and genetic factors

In particular, the Foundation lists African-Americans, Pacific Islanders and
Hispanics as being at greater risk.

The usual cycle is as follows: Person falls asleep, snoring begins,
airway begins narrowing and the person awakens with loud choking or
gasping for air. They then fall back asleep and the cycle begins all over
again.

Medical and psychological risks associated with sleep apnea include:

Increased effort to breathe in
Hypertension (high blood pressure)
Heart disease
Mood disorders
Memory problems
Drowsy driving
Heart attack
Congestive heart failure
Cardiac arrhythmia
Stroke

### *Daytime symptoms that may indicate the possibility of sleep apnea:*

Difficulty concentrating
Depression
Irritability
Sexual dysfunction
Learning and memory difficulties
Falling asleep at work, on the phone or while driving

We also go through differences in our wakefulness or sleepiness states as we age. One finding is that, as we age, we may become early-to-bed people. And it's not because of a sleep disorder, but a change in our body's needs or circadian rhythms or something yet to be discovered.

A new study points toward a possible relationship between sleep apnea and dementia. A small study of older adults aged 65 and over, who did not have cognitive impairment but had episodes of sleep apnea which were verified by their bed partners, had specific brain area scans.

The scans indicated elevated levels of a protein known as tau in the brains of those adults with obstructive sleep apnea. Tau is normally found within nerve cells and provides function and structure; however, it can also be involved in dementia.

Study subjects who had apnea had a 4.5% higher level of tau in certain portions of the brain and this raises an interesting possibility, i.e., sleep apnea may contribute to abnormal levels of tau accumulation which can result in cognitive impairment, a.k.a., dementia. But is it tau that causes apnea or apnea that somehow stimulates an abnormal level of tau in the brain?

The researchers, however, cautioned that this was a small study. Further studies are needed to replicate the finding in order to determine whether sleep apnea may cause the accumulation of tau or if there was some other indication that tau, in and of itself, causes sleep apnea.

### *Elderly, sleep apnea and cognition*

Daytime sleepiness is often reported by older adults. Many times, these individuals present with cognitive impairments and it was the opinion of one researcher that there might be an association between this and sleep-disordered breathing (SDB).

This disorder often causes excessive daytime sleepiness in the elderly. We know that being able or unable to maintain sustained, restful sleep during the night results in daytime difficulty. Then it stands to reason that frequent nighttime disruptions may result in sleepiness the next day. It is also reasonable that anyone experiencing excessive sleepiness during the day may also experience a decline in their cognitive processing.

Therefore, we should not be too hasty to jump to the conclusion that persons who are over the age of 65 would be expected to show cognitive decline. Such an expectation may result in catastrophic effects in terms of diagnosis, treatment and self-esteem.

Research found that the group with cognitive impairments had more sleep disturbances than another group which did not experience such impairments. Simple though it may seem, there is a bias that is inherent in the medical profession where older adults are assumed to experience cognitive impairment as a result of aging. Such a bias must be examined by appropriate testing before any reliable diagnosis can be made for these individuals.

The recommendation, therefore, was that any older individual who might be brought in to be screened for cognitive impairments and who was considered "elderly" should also be considered for an evaluation of a type of sleep disturbance disorder or even sleep apnea. This is not the usual procedure, however, and for that reason an important, treatable diagnosis could be missed.

The US National Institute on Aging (2012) has noted that persons over 65 should limit their alcohol intake to no more than seven drinks a week or three in one day. That is, of course, provided their treating physician agrees that alcohol will not create a medical issue.

The guidelines regarding alcohol and the elderly were issued because there was an increase in alcohol consumption in this group due to problems with sleeping, anxiety, depression or loneliness. The desire for a drink before bedtime may be in an effort to get to sleep.

### *Treatment for sleep apnea*

The treatments for this disorder always begin with a sleep study where the individual is brought into a sleep laboratory for one or two nights during which they are hooked up to monitors. Nothing painful because the sensors are taped or held in place with easily removed glue. Functions recorded by these sensors include sleep state (brain waves), eye movement, muscle activity, heart rate, respiratory effort, airflow and blood oxygen levels.

Depending on the severity of the disorder and the physical structure of the nose and throat, one of the treatments offered to patients is via a continuous positive airway pressure device (CPAP). The unit includes a face mask that fits over the nose and mouth and it provides a continuous flow of air to the person during their sleep. Many new types of these masks have come out in the past few years, so if you need one, do a bit of research.

A second approach might be the use of dental appliances. These units reposition the lower jaw and tongue. And a third approach would be surgery for the removal of excess tissue in the airway. Initially, more conservative measures would be weight loss (which can cure sleep apnea in some cases) and the avoidance of alcohol.

Alcohol, as was previously discussed, is known to cause frequent nighttime awakenings and may mimic symptoms of apnea as a result. Cigarette smoking, too, can increase swelling in the upper airway and contribute to nighttime breathing problems. A careful history is always important, and the use of alcohol and cigarettes needs to be explored.

The excessive use of alcohol by the elderly is an increasing problem noted by medical professionals. Often, again, it is overlooked and given cursory attention. Many persons who abuse alcohol will dismiss the question regarding its use with a casual remark that they "may have a glass of wine with dinner." A psychiatrist with whom I worked indicated that once you hear that, multiply it by about 4-6 and you'll probably get closer to their real consumption of alcohol.

### Narcolepsy

One note regarding another disorder that has a number of the same symptoms as sleep apnea must be made here. Narcolepsy may cause some of the same daytime or nighttime problems that include suddenly falling asleep during any activity, including sex.

There is little agreement on the cause of this disorder, but it appears to be related to a normal brain chemical (hypocretin) that is important in the regulation of the sleep/wake cycle. In those who have narcolepsy, the presence of the chemical is low and the condition is also thought to possibly be an autoimmune disorder.

Even a brain structure, the raphe, plays a potential role because it is responsible for our alertness. Other suggested causes include viral exposure to something like swine flu or genetic factors.

The usual hallmark, often, is that these sleep attacks can be brought on, without warning, by strong emotion. One good example would be as follows and which I heard at a conference.

A researcher indicated that if someone told a particularly funny joke, that person listening and laughing heartily, would suddenly fell over asleep. It can be both dangerous and frightening for all involved. Some individuals go into a state of sleep with their eyes wide open and can shift into a form of automatic action while driving a car or performing some other over-learned activity.

People have taken notes, talked on the phone or performed other actions while they were asleep. Some who have narcolepsy are totally unaware of what they had done when they later came out of the sleep state.

## *Illustrations of narcolepsy's symptoms*

At a sleep conference one woman related her experiences with narcolepsy. She commuted in a car regularly with a co-worker. The trip, where she was the driver, took them over a long, high, heavily trafficked bridge. Her friend had some considerable fear as she saw that her friend, who was driving, seemed to be in a trace, yet she continued driving the car.

The woman driver had also fallen once face down into her dinner while at a party with friends who were laughing and telling jokes. Her friends thought she had had a stroke or too much to drink. She was terribly embarrassed until she learned that she had narcolepsy. She'd suffered with the disorder for years and was often the butt of family jokes. Only after she went to a sleep lab for evaluation had she learned she did have a medical disorder. The family jokes soon stopped.

As you can see, there are clear dangers associated with this disorder since it can happen to someone who might be preparing food at a hot stove, driving a car or operating commercial machinery.

Interestingly, this sleep disorder begins to manifest itself between the ages of 10 and 25 years of age. During the years when the sleep attacks first begin ther number may be greater and then taper off a bit. Generally, it is a disorder that lasts for life, unlike sleep walking which often disappears with age.

Anyone with this type of symptomology needs to see a sleep specialist. There is no need for embarrassment.

### *Narcolepsy and REM sleep*

One interesting characteristic of these sleep attacks is that they differ from regular sleep. When we go to sleep, the usual pattern is that we begin with the cycle of non-REM (NREM) sleep that then changes later to REM (rapid eye movement) usually called the dreaming period of sleep.

But the pattern is flipped in narcolepsy where the person immediately enters REM sleep which includes a loss of muscle control and physical collapse (cataplexy), sleep paralysis and vivid hallucinations. They can literally drop to the ground without warning.

The hallucinations, which may be more properly called dreams or quasi-dreams, can be quite disturbing and frightening and lead people to think they have a mental illness. It is more than fearsome.

An additional symptom of narcolepsy is that it leaves the person feeling quite tired. This, in turn, affects their performance at work or school and they may be seen as lacking in motivation or lazy. The attacks may also lead to an expectation that they are not completely reliable and, therefore, it can affect both their ability to maintain work or to be promoted at work.

There is also an association between narcolepsy and obesity, and it is thought that a number of factors could be at work here. Suggestions include weight gain from medications, an inactive lifestyle, binge eating and a deficiency of that crucial brain hormone which functions to keep our sleep/wake cycle on track. Of all the hypothesized factors leading to narcolepsy, perhaps one presents the most interesting association with yet another recently diagnosed sleep disorder; sleep-related eating disorder.

### Sleep-related eating disorder

While those with narcolepsy may binge while awake, the patients with sleep-related eating disorder eat while sleeping. It is classified as a parasomnia, meaning an activity, apart from sleep apnea, where people do abnormal things while asleep.

Others included in this category are sleepwalking, sleep aggression and the most unusual of all, sleepsex also known as sexsomnia or SBS (somnambulistic sexual behavior) where a person engages in sex acts while totally asleep.

Sleep eating, SRED (sleep-related eating disorder) or NES (nocturnal eating syndrome), usually has a component of sleepwalking unless someone keeps a stash of food next to the bed and that doesn't seem reasonable.

The disorder can involve a number of rather complicated activities including walking to wherever the food is (usually the kitchen) and preparing a variety of foods. How complicated is the food prep? The preparation alone may present dangers to the individual and other in the home. This may happen once or several times during the night. Each time, the person eats and then returns to bed. Some patients do have a vivid memory that is like a dream to them. Others will have no memory of it at all. As you might think, it can lead to household discord.

### *Examples of sleepeating*

A fuller appreciation of just how some of the medications can affect people can be gained by listening to the patients themselves quoted in an article on zolpidem (Ambien) in the US NYU Langone Online Journal of Medicine. One man said, "I woke up sitting up in bed with a big chunk of challah bread soaked in chocolate milk in one hand and a bowl of chocolate milk in my lap. It even had ice cubes in it, the way I like it." But the activity can also include the use of sharp objects, microwaves, stoves or any other form of kitchen appliances.

A woman was startled to come face to face with her sleepeating activities as she detailed it in the following way: "I got a package of hamburger buns and I tore it open like a bear and stood there and ate the whole package." Her husband, who came upon this highly unusual scene. He said something to her and it then dawned on him that she was, indeed, asleep and totally unaware of what she was doing.

Often these types of eating disorders are noticed not only by the debris of late-night sleepeating, but also by the fact that the person's clothing is becoming tighter. Interestingly, one question that is often asked of persons who are suspected of being depressed is how their clothing fits. They may lose their appetite and never notice they're NOT eating enough during the day but eating at night as they sleep.

## Sleep and violence

Normally, sleep is a quiet time where we hopefully help ourselves get the needed rest and restoration that we need after any of our day's activities. But there are instances where sleep brings on totally unexpected circumstances which can have catastrophic results. Allow me to present you with just two instances where this did happen.

Occasional use of prescribed sleep medication, it is believed, is acceptable and within current clinical guidelines. The guidelines indicate these medications should be taken for a short course, usually seven days or less. Some individuals have chronic insomnia for which their private physicians do chronically prescribe sleep medications, and, in many cases, we never hear about bad results. But there are those times when the medication itself may, in some way, precipitate shocking actions on the part of the patient.

An example is the following case, which was ultimately a criminal one, and occurred in the western part of the United States. A middle-aged woman, who lived with her elderly mother, had an inordinate amount of stress in her life because of her caregiver responsibilities, financial difficulties and a number of other things which, together, proved to be too much for her. Her physician prescribed sleep medication which she proceeded to take over a period of years rather than days.

One morning, on her mother's 85th birthday, the woman walked into her mother's bedroom with a birthday card, a birthday cake and a loaded gun. She then proceeded to shoot her mother to death, all the while totally unaware of what she was doing. It was a type of sleep-medication-induced sleepwalking with amnesia.

The rise in the use of sleep medications, particularly problematic were the SSRI (serotonin reuptake inhibitors), was noted in 2012 in a sample of 19,136 people. Almost 30% had a lifetime prevalence of what is known as nocturnal wanderings, aka sleepwalking behavior while taking these medications.

A family history of such behavior was reported in just over 30%. This is noted as somewhat high and was thought to be related to individuals with a prior history of major depressive disorder (MDD) or obsessive-compulsive disorder (OCD).

The chronic use of sleep medications, too, bears watching. We do know that such medications can cause short-term amnesia for the following day and, for that reason, a number of European countries have banned certain dosages of sleep medications.

Another case in point in Europe involved a young physician who was going to attend a day-long seminar. The woman took the medication the night before a meeting, woke up the next morning, went to the seminar for the entire day and later could remember nothing of what she did or said during the entire day. It was a complete blank. She was not alone in experiencing this type of amnesia even though she didn't take the medication on a daily basis.

Back to the woman in the western United States. She was arrested for her mother's murder but was found not guilty because she was severely impaired by a sleep syndrome that was caused, her attorney successfully argued, by her medication. After she was released from police custody, she filed a major lawsuit against the pharmaceutical company and her physician, and she did win her case.

There are other times, however, when violence during sleep is not related to a medication, but rather, experts tell us, to a specific type of nocturnal epilepsy or other form of sleep disorder. The name they have given to this is sleep-related violence (SRV) and another involving sex is sexual behavior in sleep (SBS).

While in this state, these individuals can act out violently toward others to the point of causing major physical harm to someone or damage to furniture in the room where they are sleeping. One man threw a bedroom dresser through the window and began violently punching his wife and had no memory later. Sometimes, without proper diagnosis and treatment, these individuals when married find themselves headed to divorce court.

Sleep violence has been reported since the Middle Ages and even the very famous creator of therapeutic hypnosis, Charcot, told of a man who, while in a sleepwalking state, attempted to murder two individuals with a gun.

Usually, sleepwalking is not associated with violence and the only danger is that the individual who is sleepwalking may harm themselves by tripping or falling down a flight of stairs. One man did find himself standing on a roof during the middle of the night. He had no idea how he got there because all he recalled was that he went to bed and fell asleep.

Unusual, and we might say criminal behavior, has also been reported in the literature where sexual assaults have been perpetrated on minors. A small study of only 31 patients reported that 45% displayed assaultive behavior relative to their sleep disorder. There were legal charges that could be lodged against these individuals.

Researchers refers to these disorders as a form of nocturnal epilepsy or R.E.M. Sleep Behavior Disorder (RBD). Generally, the individuals have some type of dream activity going on which is threatening and where they must defend themselves. In a state of semi-arousal, they are out of bed and attempting to attack these imaginary dangers. The "dangers", of course, are those who happened to be in the room with them and who are, most probably, sleeping soundly.

Studies have evaluated the incidence of sleep-related harmful behavior but, unfortunately, the samples used were small and the results are questionable. Some have indicated that 2% of the population is prone to this disorder but this has been seen as unreliable data.

We do know, however, that it is more common in males over the age of 50 than females and that it may run in families. Another interesting finding is that scientists have located lesions in an area of the brainstem that would usually inhibit physical movement during sleep. A lesion such as this may liberate nighttime activity during sleep and bring on this behavior.

Should anyone you know be engaging in sleep-related troubling actions or aggression, there is no doubt that a professional referral must be considered. No one wants anyone to be hurt while they're awake or asleep and not getting help is, to put it mildly, dangerous.

There's no shame in having this type of sleep-related disorder. It's a medical condition just like any other medical condition for which you would seek treatment.

# CHAPTER 10

# Sleep-related Physical Problems

◆ ◆ ◆

*Men who are unhappy, like men who sleep badly,*
*are always proud of the fact. - Bertrand Russell*

Sleep deprivation exacts more than a measure of impairment on our mental capacity because it is intimately involved in our physical functioning as well. The disorders, parts of the body and diseases that may be associated with sleep deprivation can seem more than alarming once you begin to delve into them.

With so many Americans developing the autoimmune disorder of diabetes, including children, we are always being exhorted to eat less, watch what we eat and exercise more. There's an emphasis on cutting down on our sugar and salt intake, but sleep is NEVER mentioned as an important component of a healthy lifestyle plan.

Where is the mention of getting a sufficient number of hours of sleep each day? Again, it's among the missing when it comes to advice on how to remain healthy.

In fact, we probably rely too much on our healthcare professionals to keep us informed. I'm not saying they don't know their own specialties, but an illustration might be helpful here.

I once had a job where I was involved in assisting pharmaceutical firms market their products and we had to do a bit of research because one of the items tasked to us was for weight control. Everyone knows how important weight control is and it's a multi-million-dollar, if not multi-billion-dollar field. The fight against fat is a continuing one.

In order to prepare a presentation for one of our clients and pitch a one-million-dollar program to them, I decided we needed to know how much time was spent in medical education on diet and nutrition. Aren't we constantly being told to ask our physicians about diet?

I contacted 12 major medical schools in the United States and requested information on the number of hours spent by medical students in learning about diet and nutrition. Know how many hours they received on average, if they got any at all? Just about one or two hours in a lecture-type setting without any handouts or very much discussion in a Q&A format was all the education they received on the subject. After hearing this, how informed do you suppose most of those physicians were?

Who knows better than you about sleep? Does your regular physician, that you visit either regularly or for an annual physical, ask about sleep? Makes sense, doesn't it that this person should guide you.

## Alzheimer's and sleep

One large sample of older nuns (Snowdon, 2008) found that increased education and continuing lifelong learning appeared to ward off Alzheimer's dementia. The study, which began in 1986, is one of the longest running research projects on ageing and Alzheimer's.

One of the nuns lived to 105 and was still cognitively intact at her death. The day before she died, she was crocheting booties for babies in the local hospital. Sleep was not, to my knowledge, one of the factors studied in that research, either.

The nuns who were least cognitively impaired and who lived longest, interestingly, were those who over the course of their lives maintained a positive attitude toward their lives. Some nuns made it a regular target for each new year to learn some new skill or a language.

We know that being positive can also affect sleep, but the study didn't (so far) provide evidence of how these nuns' sleep patterns may have differed. Sleep can contribute to better mood and that affects our outlook on life. I'm assuming that the nuns were sound sleepers who got a sufficient amount of sleep to bolster their mood.

New research evidence has pointed to a particularly interesting association between sleep and Alzheimer's Disease. A study performed at the University of California San Diego suggested there was a disruption of the normal sleep rhythm (circadian rhythm disruption or SCRD). Patients in the early stages of the disorder who manifested these changes in sleep patterns were found to have a sped-up progression of Alzheimer's in terms of the formation of brain-damaging plaques seen in Alzheimer's.

The connection between sleep and the immune system has been well-established at this point. Further research involving those with a sleep disorder not related to sleep apnea found that lack of sleep was involved, in some manner, in rheumatoid arthritis, ankylosing spondylitis, systemic lupus erythematosus, Sjogren's syndrome, and systemic sclerosis.

Persons with a sleep disorder were found to be at higher risk of developing an autoimmune disorder and, once again, the connection was heightened in terms of its dangerous predisposition to these serious disorders. Sleep disturbance has also been found to be associated with inflammatory disease risk and recent research has indicated that this finding is global in nature.

We can rule out many of the other factors that we would consider and be pretty confident that the culprit appears to be sleep restriction. We also know that stress can play a role in inflammatory diseases and autoimmune disorders and it would seem practical to suggest that lack of sleep increases daytime stress.

Daytime stress then has a deleterious feedback effect on the body and the cycle of sleep deprivation begins. Hunting for other causes before ruling out sleep deprivation would seem to be hasty when the evidence may be right there waiting for the asking. And dismissing daytime stress as a contributory factor isn't wise, either.

## Blood pressure

Do you have hypertension, a.k.a. high blood pressure? There may be a number of reasons for it and one of them is constant stress. At this point, you already know that the stress hormone, cortisol, can get out of control when you're stressed, and sleep deprived.

Of course, stress leads to difficulty in getting to sleep and frequent insomnia, so there's a good reason to believe that your BP leaves you exposed to stroke, problems in your kidneys, in circulation in the limbs, and, if left untreated and sufficiently high, the ultimate price is paid. Ratings on BP of high-stressed individuals who may also lack sleep because of the stress are going to be higher than normal. What might be an alternative to medication?

A major study of over 10,000 persons in China found that there was a direct association between multiple factors of poor sleep quality, short sleep duration, prolonged inability to get to sleep and sleep disturbances and an increased odds of developing hypertension.

The studies like this one, again, have stressed the importance of sleep as a major factor in health.

## Cancer

The World Health Organization has viewed sleep loss as not only an epidemic worldwide but has indicated nighttime shiftwork is a probably cause of cancer in nightshift workers and is a carcinogen. Night shift workers are working against the body's natural circadian rhythm and because of this the body is not able to engage in its normal repair, restoration and preparation for the next day. It is also using up resources which you would normally be using for vital body maintenance during the night. How might it be affecting the development of cancers?

One study, where subjects were permitted to sleep only six hours a night for one week, indicated that almost 700 genes in our body were affected by sleep deprivation. Half of the genes were involved in immune function. Their ability to function was depressed while the other half, which was involved in tumor promoting, inflammation and cardiovascular disease, saw an uptick in their activity.

This striking indication of sleep as being involved, at the genetic level, was totally unexpected. One sleep expert indicated that sleep-deprived people place themselves at risk of dying from heart disease because scientists have noticed this decreased ability to protect us, in terms of our genes, and the increase in markers for inflammation. It is his opinion that if we get less than six hours sleep a night, we risk our mortality. When did we ever think lack of sleep would result in a short lifespan because of cancer?

## Dementia and excessive sleep?

Is there such a thing as sleeping too much and does it have significant diagnostic indicators for dementia? The question was posed by recent research by Westwood et al. (2016) where the team sought to tease out if there might be a risk of "incident dementia" and a relationship to brain aging.

The well-known Framingham Heart Study data was used to analyze self-reports of total hours of sleep in 2,457 patients with a mean age of 72 (57% were women). They also delved into the questions of risk of dementia over 10 years as well as brain volume and performance on cognitive testing.

In all, 234 cases, of what they termed "all-cause dementia," were found over the 10-year follow-up period. It should be noted that there was also an association with a less-than-high-school level of education in subjects who were more likely to sleep for 9 hours and had six times the risk for dementia. This is pretty disquieting and may or may not be helpful in diagnosing early dementia via neurodegeneration, aka cell death.

There have been contradictory results found on a number of sleep studies with older adults. Some found that shorter sleepers (those getting 6 hours or less) were more prone to dementia. Here, we see the opposite, but this re-analysis looked at the same individuals over a 13-year period, so they had two end points to compare sleep and cognition. Few other studies had such robust material with which to work and, therefore, to formulate some speculative results.

One problem with this analysis, which the researchers admit, was that there may have been problems in the calculation and self-reported cognition at the beginning of the study. Although easy to obtain, self-report is always challenging because few of us can provide accurate information regarding ourselves.

We're all biased; some in a negative manner, some in a more positive frame. Outside validation of the reports weren't available, so the data was entered as it came in. Most researchers, unfortunately, are just happy to get the data and to move their studies along.

One question, which I would pose, is whether the brains of these long-sleepers were desperately trying to clean up debris and not being successful. Their brains were lighter in cerebral weight, too, which may have meant that the damage was already done and couldn't be reversed by cleaning.

But where, along the horizontal axis of years, could some remediation have been successful via, possibly, extra sleep in terms of naps or longer nighttime sleeping? Intriguing questions, especially if just getting more sleep could have proven to be an answer to a serious problem in a large growing group of adults.

Not wanting to stray into a too-technical area here, I might also ask if regular collection of white blood cell counts were made. These cells tell us about inflammation and "cleaners" present to help with natural housekeeping. In another area, education was an issue.

Many in the sample didn't have a high school education. Were they not engaged in some type of continued learning, be it taking up a hobby, a part-time job or anything else where new learning would be acquired? The issue here is that lifelong learning, as you now know, is important in keeping our minds agile as our bodies are helped by regular exercise.

Wouldn't it be wonderful if we could see not only sleep, but part-time employment for older adults, as a health benefit? Why wouldn't insurance companies offer lower premiums to people who did both, if we had the research to support this?

Here's another doctoral dissertation just waiting for someone with the sharpness to recognize a viable topic when one falls into their lap. I once did offer a suggestion for an extension on an Alzheimer's protocol where I saw that social interaction, within the family and outside of it, was something important to measure in terms of a medication's efficacy.

Yes, a student picked up on my question and did a dissertation, but I was somewhat shocked that the original researchers hadn't looked into that aspect of their study and hadn't put in place some means of measuring it. They were too focused on the biology and forgot the psychology part of anything to do with mental health or cognition.

For the researchers, it would have been as simple as a patient beginning to say, "Good morning" after taking a few doses of the medication. It was an incidental finding that would have been lost if not for that student picking it up after I mentioned it in a study conference.

### Diabetes

Buy all the Lean Cuisine, Weight Watchers or whoever's meals you want but if you're not sleeping, you're sweeping the ocean back with a dust broom. And the more you diet, you may find the harder it becomes to lose weight, especially as you get older. One of the most convincing studies of the connection between diabetes and sleep deprivation was facilitated by the Nurses' Health Study, a data-collection study that ran from 1976 through 1989.

Women, who didn't have diabetes, cardiovascular disease or cancer by the year 2000, were involved. The study is impressive not only for the results but for the fact that the nurses remained in it for 10 years.

What were the findings? An astounding 6,407 of them reported they had been diagnosed with type II diabetes during that 10-year period. Sleep problems either falling asleep or remaining asleep, were reported by almost 5 percent of the women in the second half of the study (it was run in two phases). The researchers then discovered that 45% of the women who had frequent trouble sleeping were more likely to develop type II diabetes than those who didn't have sleep problems.

When the data was further analyzed, two or more sleep disturbances were discovered; sleep apnea or sleeping fewer than six hours a night. Those nurses with a lack of restful sleep had a four-fold increase in risk for developing type II diabetes. Sleep disturbance, the researchers concluded, was an important contributor to this autoimmune disorder and also an important means of preventing the disorder.

Their final conclusion in just this one study, and there are many other studies that have replicated the results in shorter time frames, was that, *"Sleep difficulty was significantly associated with type II diabetes. This association was partially explained by associations with hypertension, BMI (body mass index) and depression symptoms and was particularly strong when combined with other sleep disorders…"*

A second study by Van Coulter et al. (2005) reviewed not only sleep deprivation and hormones, but metabolism and also made a case for how our 24-hours-a-day society contributed to the development of physical disorders. Indications in this study point to sleep having a marked influence over what is known as the master gland, the pituitary.

It is well known, they indicated, that "*sleep loss is associated with an increase in appetite that is excessive in relation to the caloric demands of extended wakefulness.*" This is quite an interesting connection and may point to why persons who have sleep deprivation also are struggling with weight gain related to appetite increase.

For anyone interested in pursuing some reading on this connection, be sure to take a look at how sleep restriction affects our body's production of the hormone known as leptin that is believed to control appetite. Of course, researchers had discovered the leptin connection to appetite and hoped to design a medication to control it, but that hasn't happened. Perhaps, it's a good thing because sleep may be the course of first resort rather than pharmaceuticals.

If sleep and stress are important determents of your health, what might happen if you failed to consider steps to insure you get adequate sleep and work toward reducing stress? Read on.

## Exercise and muscle strength

Another sleep study looked at the intriguing connection between sleep duration and not dementia but muscle strength via measures of hand strength (Chen et al., 2017). The results of this study, carried out in Taiwan, show that there seemed to be a relationship between decreased hand grip strength (aka muscle strength in general) and longer sleep duration. Were the muscles responsible for longer or shorter sleep and did exercise play a role here? Fascinating thoughts to ponder.

Wouldn't it be interesting if exercise and building up or maintaining muscle strength could, in some way, affect rates of dementia shown in sleep duration? It would seem a logical piece of new research or an extension of this one.

Do elderly who exercise rigorously express slower rates of cognitive decline and could a program of exercise be a potential treatment for early decline and also provide positive results in terms of quality of sleep and length of sleep? Again, good questions and I hope they're being asked somewhere.

One study, in a sea of plenty, which viewed a relationship between exercise and cognitive decline in older adults (Behrman & Ebmeier, 2014) did find that dancing or any physical form of exercise provided results not dissimilar to medication when it came to depression.

This research team had indicated that exercise is also useful in fostering self-esteem, warding off negative thoughts and improving what is known as executive function, or decision making. Wouldn't there be other positive findings?

If self-esteem is improved and negative thoughts are held at bay, it stands to reason that sleep duration or quality of sleep could also benefit. Sleep was not included in factors they evaluated during this particular study.

The research, however, would seem to be getting closer to the association between a variety of factors associated with sleep and cognition. But another study raised interesting questions about activities of daily living. The results are not in yet but it will be of great interest to all of us.

## Heart attacks and sleep loss

It's understandable that sometimes you can't get the sleep you need, but don't skimp on it. One time when over *one billion people* all together experience a form of sleep deprivation is during changes in *daylight saving time*. The literature has shown that an analysis of 42,000 admissions to a heart attack unit at a hospital in the United States between 2010 and 2013 revealed that there was a *24% increase in heart attack* admissions on the *Monday after daylight saving time* change. Interestingly, when the clocks were turned back again in the fall to the be in sync with the original time, there was a *21% decrease in heart attacks* on *the Tuesday following this change.*

In other words, people were getting that extra hour of sleep and were not being deprived of sleep. Can we say that sleep deprivation of only one hour would produce such drastic results in the incidence of heart attacks? No, not positively but the incidence of heart attacks must be seen as a further indicator of the hidden dangers for people who are sleep deprived.

## Immune system killer cells

Our bodies protect themselves by the ceaseless activity of what we know as "killer cells" or our T cells. These masterful bits of material form our internal army, ever ready to fight off the attacks of viruses and bacteria. Infection is their primary enemy and they do it relentlessly day and night—but only with a bit of help from you. What do they require to be most efficient? Putting it simply, it's sleep.

How important is sleep to the functioning of these killers? After getting only four hours of sleep for one night, studies have shown a 70% drop in natural killer cell activity. An astonishing decrease like that should concern anyone about their health. The lack of a robust immune killer cell army is seen as being behind the increases in cancer of the bowel, the prostate and the breast.

## Inflammatory disease

A review (Irwin, 2016) of extensive research over the past several decades provided an analysis of 72 research reports on a total of 50,000 participants. These participants were from both population-based as well as clinical-trial studies.

The reports, the researchers concluded, showed that both in the population-based studies as well as the clinical trials, there was a relationship between getting too little sleep as well as too much sleep. Both of these conditions resulted in increased inflammatory levels. Getting the right amount of sleep, therefore, is essential.

The researchers found definitive clinical markers for levels of inflammatory indicators in the blood of study participants in both groups. The markers are linked with chronic diseases such as heart problems, hypertension and type II diabetes. They suggest that poor sleep is associated with these inflammatory processes.

Therefore, in addition to diet and exercise, sleep plays a vital role in the control of inflammation in a number of chronic conditions and in the stress hormone, cortisol.

If you find this a bit unusual, I must agree with you because we would suspect that getting too little sleep, a.k.a. sleep deprivation, would be the culprit in inflammatory processes. The research studies, however, also find too much sleep is involved in this inflammatory process which would seem to be a contradiction. However, the inflammatory markers make the case for a system that is somewhat askew with what would be expected.

An earlier study in 2015 also found inflammation associated with too little or too much sleep. This study, however, indicated that there was an additional risk of depression as well as diabetes. The information we're receiving from all of these studies, whether they chose people from off the street or in clinical trials, is pointing to something we cannot ignore. The evidence supports a connection between inflammation in asthma, inflammatory bowel disease, rheumatoid arthritis, and even certain forms of cancer.

The finding of inflammation in depression was one which the researchers found particularly interesting. They believe more investigation needs to be conducted in this particular link with inflammation and lack of sleep.

Gestational diabetes mellitus found in pregnancy has also been studied (2017) in a multi-ethnic Asian population. Sleep was identified as one of the main factors involved in high levels of glucose metabolism in those who had problems sleeping. An interesting side note was provided by the researchers who indicated that adults living in Singapore, where this research study was conducted, are among the most sleep-deprived adults in the world.

## Jet lag

But how about people who have to travel a great deal and experience jet lag on a regular basis? This, too, has been addressed by researchers in sleep. Traveling over long distances that, in effect, artificially tried to reset our internal clock, isn't going to work. We know that sleep timing plays a vital factor in physical functioning.

Laboratory studies that mimicked this type of jet lag result showed an imbalance in glucose metabolism and we know that is associated with type II diabetes. It can only be assumed that chronic jet lag will have some residual physical effects. Whether these can be ameliorated by some type of sleep restoration upon return to one's home base, is a matter to be further studied.

The researchers had an interesting name for jet lag and they called it *"living against the clock."* They did see it as a real contributor to weight–related pathologies and, in turn, that could mean changes to the physical health of anyone with this "against the clock" schedule. How could it not be otherwise?

The stress hormone, cortisol, is one that is closely associated with sleep and, in fact, its level in your body rises during the night. Travel of any kind is stressful enough so imagine that you are also sleep deprived and functioning against your biological clock. The result cannot be good for you.

## Perceptual changes

After a sleepless or night of fitful sleep, we are not only fatigued but there are apparent perceptual changes which result in our having a more negative interpretation of things in our lives. We are short-tempered and may be prone to an increase in depression as well as what was deemed a "negative bias."

This bias results in a gloomy interpretation of interactions with others and potential interpersonal or job dysfunction. At home it could cause family discord, but in the office, it could cost you your job.

## Pregnancy and Sleep

Pregnancy, as every mother knows, bring with a plethora of delights and a number of physical changes, one of them being disturbances in sleep. Both physiological and psychological aspects of pregnancy can bring on sleep deprivation in women and it has been stated that insomnia during pregnancy remains largely underdiagnosed.

The problem of sleep disorders in pregnancy is not that it is a discomfort for the woman, so much as it carries with it the possibility of physical illness for her and also for the growing fetus. It has been determined that women who experience sleep deprivation during their pregnancy may give birth to children that have cognitive developmental issues.

The developing fetus is particularly vulnerable during these periods of sleep deprivation because in addition to the possibility of developing an anxiety disorder, these children may also develop learning disabilities and ADHD. The World Health Organization (WHO) has estimated that 10% of currently pregnant women and 13% who have just given birth have children who show the development of mental disorders *as a result of maternal sleep disorders*. According to a number of researchers, maternal sleep deprivation has been understudied and is a vital issue which needs to be addressed. WHO has indicated that it is one of their major concerns outside of malnutrition.

### *Insomnia, restless legs and sleep apnea*

The most notable changes in terms of sleep disorders in pregnant women have been in the areas of:

restless legs syndrome (aka gRLS which varies from 10-38% of pregnancies)
obstructive sleep apnea
narcolepsy
insomnia
numbers of physical disorders such as hypertension and diabetes related to the pregnancy.

In an internet-based study of slightly over 2,400 women, the researchers indicated the following sleep-related problems of pregnant women. In that study, the list of problems are patient-centered complaints rather than diagnostic sleep disorders and were:

100% indicated frequent nighttime awakenings
76% experienced poor-quality sleep (less REM sleep)
57% reported Insomnia
49% complained of daytime sleepiness
38% said that they had insufficient sleep time
24% reported restless leg syndrome (gestational RLs or gRLS)
19% had sleep disordered breathing

Breathing disorders, especially obstructive sleep apnea (OSA) has been found in several studies and is associated with gestational weight gain and plays a significant role in hypertension during pregnancy. The OSA is seen as associated with physical changes which are pregnancy-related such as nasal congestion, pharyngeal edema, tracheal shortening and abdominal mass with decreased lung volume. All of this underscores the seriousness of OSA in these women and the need for appropriate professional treatment.

Women with higher body mass indexes (BMIs) are more likely to experience chronic hypertension as shown in one study where 55.6% of them exhibited this potentially serious problem. OSA has also been implicated as precipitating not only hypertension but unplanned delivery, preterm births, admission to neonatal intensive care units or special-care nurseries, cesarean delivery and gestational diabetes.

The sleep disorder, RLS (Restless Legs Syndrome), which is predominant in females, shows a 2-3-fold increase during pregnancy possibly related to changes in neural hormones as well as changes in iron. Women with a family history of RLS are much more likely to experience it during their pregnancy and it may be mild to moderate in nature. Severe RLS, however, has been reported in some cases.

The possibility of developing gRLS has been viewed as related to the risk factors of smoking, snoring in the first trimester and obesity. In fact, women who experienced gRLS were twice as likely to also have pregnancy-induced hypertension (PIH) and scored significantly higher on the Epworth Sleepiness Scale. These women were seen as significantly at higher risk for perinatal depression.

Insomnia during pregnancy was also a concern because of the dysfunction in their daytime activities. While chronic insomnia may occur in 10% of the population, transient insomnia in pregnant women is between 30-35% and this occurs primarily during the first trimester. However, in one study of 370 pregnant women, insomnia worsened during the third trimester as scored by the Insomnia Severity Index (*see Appendix C*). Overall, study researchers indicated that the greater majority of pregnant women (73.5%) had insomnia at some time during their pregnancy.

A curious finding, however, was reported in one study of pregnant women and insomnia. Twenty-two percent of the women in the study reported eating at night. This was three times higher in women who developed insomnia. Problems in the research protocol's failure to follow up on this finding, however, make this difficult to assess. Did they eat because they were experiencing insomnia or because they were hungry or because they had a pre-existing sleep disorder where persons eat while still sleeping?

In terms of treatment for insomnia during pregnancy, professionals advise nonpharmacologic treatments, sleep hygiene as well as cognitive-behavior therapy. Acupuncture has also been shown to increase the body's natural sleep-inducing substance, melatonin. When compared to women in a sleep-hygiene group, those receiving acupuncture had decreases in their insomnia scores of 50-75%. The small size of the study, however, is reason to view it with caution and requires further exploration of this modality as an effective treatment for this particular type of insomnia.

Regarding pregnant women who work, there has been some evidence of a circadian sleep-wake disorder (CSWD) which may have an effect on gestational age, low birth-weight babies, preterm delivery and fetal loss. Although not specifically studied in pregnancy, there have been studies in the general population that indicate the utility of using full-spectrum white light or blue or green light for CSWD. This light application is used at specific times during the person's normal circadian cycle and may manage the disorder.

Researchers also suggest scheduled naps as well as consistency in bedtime and arising as well, the latter being an important component of a sleep hygiene program. However, researchers also know, for some as-yet-unknown reason, a pregnant woman's natural circadian rhythm is changed during the first trimester.

The result is that their daily schedules are shifted earlier by several hours. They have noted that prior research has pointed to shiftwork as one of the factors involved in this disruptive shift. Thus far, there has been inadequate exploration of the causes that may be contributing to this shift which can have important implications for births and the delivery of the child.

## Sexual health in men

A Danish study of 953 young men was conducted to explore the association between sleep disturbance, serum sperm quality, testosterone level and testicle size. Measures of sleep disturbance were taken and those with a high level of sleep disturbance showed a 29% lower sperm concentration and fewer normal sperm cells than men with a lower sleep disturbance score. The researchers indicate that this association between sleep and disturbances in sperm quality is of special note and, again, requires additional research.

In today's highly industrialized world, we are in a period of sperm quality decline which has been reported in the literature. One week of sleep restriction to five hours a night in one study resulted in a *10 to 15% decrease in testosterone levels*. Another study of 531 Chinese men found that longer sleep durations increased testosterone level but the researchers indicate the findings could not be confirmed. But the question of men's sexual health and sleep requires serious consideration and more study.

Not only were there several differences in measures of sperm and testosterone, but testicle size was also significantly lower in men who had higher sleep deprivation scores. Poor sleep was seen in a reduction of sperm concentration of 25% fewer normal sperm cells.

Numerous researchers have indicated that stress may play an issue and that there may be multiple factors including lack of sleep in fertility rates as it relates to men. The levels of testosterone found in sleep-deprived young men, however, were those that would have been expected in older men. Sleep would appear to be a culprit in one of several factors in these decreases in significant terms of male sexuality.

A study of healthy young college man recruited for a one-week sleep study also indicated results in changing testosterone level. The men who slept less than five hours a night for one week had significantly lower levels of testosterone than those who had a full night's sleep. Low levels of testosterone have been equated with negative mood changes in sexual behavior and reproduction, critical changes in strength and muscle mass in addition to bone density. Also significant was the students' level of vigor which was noted immediately after the completion of the study. Their vigor continued to fall each day after the five-hours-of-sleep trials. The effect, therefore, was not limited and continued to show mood and stamina decreases for some time afterward.

One researcher, Dr. Eve Van Cauter, indicated that 15% of the adult male population in the US gets less than five hours sleep a night. Skipping sleep reduces a man's testosterone level by the equivalent of aging them *10 to 15 years older* than their current age. Normally, testosterone levels in males will decline by 1 to 2% a year beginning in a man's late 30s, but this research showed a dramatic and sleep-related change in young, healthy males.

## Sleep and the kidneys

Some of us think we can just catch up on the weekend and things will be fine, but our bodies don't always agree with that route to health and reduction of sleep debt. Researchers have reasoned that after four or five nights of less sleep, we can catch up on the weekend with a few extra hours in bed.

But you can't keep doing that. Sooner or later those weekends sleeping in don't do the job and your immune system may be the first part of your body to take note. You will then find you are getting more colds, more prone to the flu or your blood glucose level is off. The pancreas is not functioning normally and that is one serious endocrine gland. Also, your kidneys may start to have problems. Who would think that lack of sleep could be what has been deemed the "gateway to kidney dysfunction?"

According to a research report from Brigham and Women's Hospital in Boston that was quoted in WebMD, "women who slept five hours or less a night had a 65% greater risk of rapid decline in kidney function, compared with women sleeping 7 to 8 hours a night…" The study was fairly robust and involved 4,238 nurses whereas many studies may have fewer than 100 or so. This finding can't be ignored.

One of the main researchers, McMullen, cautioned that they couldn't make a case that less sleep causes kidney damage, but it is associated with it. His team theorizes, however, that less sleep may change the kidneys' physiology in some way, and this leads to damage.

## Sleep and pain

One of the most interesting aspects of sleep is that it serves as a natural pain killer because there is a center within the brain that gauges pain sensitivity as it relates to sleep. Inadequate sleep or sleep deprivation appears to increase our sensitivity to pain by numbing this particular brain center and putting the brakes on what is a natural mechanism for relieving pain.

The brain center responsible for monitoring pain signals throughout the body and preparing an appropriate reaction to tamp down pain sensitivity is known as the brain's insula and it is underactive during periods of sleep deprivation. One researcher, obviously expressing how helpful he felt this brain center was, called it nature's painkiller and saw it as a means to decrease pain through adequate sleep.

The Centers for Disease Control and Prevention (CDC) have indicated that 20% of the American population, or about 50 million adults, live with chronic pain and in attempting to alleviate this pain, the result is about 130 people die every day from an overdose of pain medication. Sleep, therefore, would appear to provide a safe alternative to pain medications.

The finding of a sleep-pain connection is not a new one. Research over the past several decades has shown a positive relationship between sleep deprivation, in some instances of only one night, and the sensation of painful osteoarthritis, fibromyalgia and chronic migraine headaches. The conclusion that can be drawn from this vast trove of material is that sleep definitely plays a vital role in pain relief.

## Sleep and suicide

Suicide, while intensely studied over the past century, remains a significant health problem worldwide and in some instances, approximately 40,000 Americans will commit suicide in any one year. One factor which has not been studied closely is the involvement of sleep or insomnia in suicide deaths until 25 years ago when the first research article on this association appeared in professional journals.

Several factors are involved in suicide as it pertains to sleep and they include the fact that that the lack of sleep prevents normal cognitive functioning during the daytime, interferes with the ability to make rational decisions and can increase feelings of hopelessness and depression. Therefore, researchers are beginning to understand that exploring whether or not someone is experiencing sleep disturbances must be a question for anyone who is either depressed or expressing suicidal thinking.

Understandably, the inability to sleep restfully can bring on a degree of hopelessness and this will only compound existing problems. It is also believed that there may be some differences in what sleep provides or, rather, what it disrupts and that may be important neurotransmitters in the brain which are involved in our thinking processes and our emotions.

Insomnia has also been deemed a state of hyper arousal where the person is agitated and unable to rest and this may require medical intervention, however, there may also be methods for helping persons with this type of agitation that are not pharmacologic. The research so far indicates that the association between sleep disturbance and suicide has been found all over the world and includes children, adolescents, young adults and the elderly.

An article in *The Psychiatric Times* indicated that "*...the increasing evidence for sleep disturbance as a suicide risk factor, and possible warning sign, have led researchers to explore for mechanisms behind the association of sleep disturbance and suicide. This research, still in its infancy, has the potential to improve our understanding of the contexts in which sleep disturbances confer increased risk for suicide.*

*Dissatisfaction with the quality, timing, and duration of sleep, as well as the subsequent distress or impairment during waking hours, are considered typical manifestations across all sleep-wake disorders. It is not clear if such dissatisfaction or impairment can uniformly explain why those with sleep problems are at increased risk for attempting suicide. It has been hypothesized, however, that difficulty sleeping through the night may confer increased suicide risk via a number of factors including hyperarousal, hypothalamic-pituitary-adrenal (HPA) axis dysfunction, and concomitant serotonin dysfunction.*"

### *Teen sleep and suicide*

Sleep deprivation, especially when it is found in adolescents, must be taken seriously as having the potential for life-taking behaviors. An advisory in *Psychiatric News* should provide enough grim information to be truly disturbing. It states:

"*Among U.S. adolescents, suicide is second only to unintentional injury (chiefly involving motor vehicles) as the leading cause of death. In*

*2016, the most recent year for which the CDC provides statistics, 2,553 youths aged 10 to 19 years died of suicide in this country.*" An analysis provides some insight into the activities which may be precipitated by sleep deprivation and they include engaging in *higher risk-taking behavior, use of alcohol, smoking and driving while drunk.*"

One specific study in Fairfax County, VA, in the US evaluated the relationship between sleep deprivation and school-start times. The conclusions offer some areas of particular note and specific groups which may be more prone to suicide related to their sleep deprivation. The researchers stated:

*"We identified certain groups in this study that interventionists should perhaps monitor more closely with respect to sleep and suicide: (a) female teens, who sleep less in general and are already at increased risk for depression, (b) Asian teens, who are the most sleep deprived and for whom amount of sleep appears particularly important in predicting suicidality, and (c) males with reduced sleep who appear to be most susceptible to actual suicidal attempts. The current study also suggests that sleep continues to be important for predicting teen suicidality independent of its role in teen depression, suggesting that adults need to continue to monitor and facilitate teen sleep even after knowledge that their adolescent is depressed.*"

Adequate sleep for children and teens is so important for daytime functioning, academic performance and attending school on time that the American Academy of Sleep Medicine (AASM) has recommended that schools start later rather than earlier in order to assist children and teens in getting a full night sleep.

In concert with the AASM, the Centers for Disease Control indicates that waking children up later, again, provides them with the more than seven hours of sleep which they require. Interestingly, it has been noted that during childhood and puberty the sleep-inducing hormone *melatonin is produced on a delayed schedule*. This release change in children results in their not being tired before 11 PM at night. Therefore, they may spend time in bed and not be asleep until after 11 and when they have to wake up before 7:30 AM they are not getting sufficient sleep.

Schools that start classes before 8 AM in the morning are, in effect, providing fuel to the fire in that they are causing chronic sleep loss which is associated with poor school performance, higher risk for depression, obesity, cardiovascular problems, risk-taking behavior and athletic injuries. Of course, there are other consequences, too, but these are of primary consideration.

A study that was published in the Journal of Clinical Sleep Medicine found that automobile crash rates fell by 16.5% in the two-year period after schools shifted to a later start time when compared to two years prior to that shift. Think of how many lives or injuries could have been avoided by a change in school start times.

Schools across the country, when planning their school year calendars, should take the research regarding sleep deprivation in students into consideration. Of course, not everyone is in agreement and there have been comments that it is the parents and not the school time that is responsible for poor academic performance and unacceptable behavior.

Parents can play a vital role in the amount of sleep that their children get. To facilitate better sleep schedules and better-quality sleep, there are a number of steps that have been recommended. Some of these include:

not allowing the use of technology in the bedroom
parents setting a good example by reading a book at bedtime
spending more time together as a family

Consider the early start time that many schools have instituted and then consider how difficult this is for a child who has not had 8 to 10 hours, or at least seven hours, of quality sleep. If school starts at 7:35 AM, the kids must be on the bus most probably at 6:45 AM and must have awakened by 6 AM in order to get ready. In order to work at their best efficiency, children would have to be asleep by no later than 10 PM. However, the recommended number of hours of sleep is eight – 10. Experts admit that it would be a difficult task to have teenagers in bed and asleep by 10 o'clock at night, however.

It has been estimated that 80% of middle and high schools in the United States have not abided by these research-based recommendations for later starts for school classes. The majority, therefore, continue to promote early start times. In the face of science, they have chosen otherwise, and children are sleep-deprived as a result.

One of the most striking findings in an analysis of data from almost 68,000 high school students was that students who got fewer hours of sleep were more likely to engage in unsafe behavior. High school students who slept less than six hours are twice as likely to use a variety of drugs or driving after drinking.

One of the most serious findings of research is that short sleep duration was strongly associated with mood and self-harm and those students who got less than six hours of sleep typically were three times as likely to feel sad, hopeless, seriously considered suicide, had a plan to attempt suicide or had attempted suicide. In fact, they were *four times as likely to have a suicide attempt* that required treatment when compared to students who slept eight hours or more at night. In all, 23,000 students reported depressed mood and seriously considered or attempted suicide.

## Sleep hygiene education of physicians

Was it because there was too much other material to learn in medical school or was this something the schools didn't' feel could be fit into their curriculum? Who knows? All I knew was that the physicians were woefully lacking in this knowledge. How much training do you suppose medical students get on sleep? Probably they're told to send patients to a sleep center and that's not a bad idea, but what about some easy-to-manage information on sleep hygiene?

I see regular press releases on how food will now be labeled with the caloric content, restaurants will provide us with all manner of nutritional information and celebrities are going to join the business to get the obese in line. Diabetes, we're being told, is an epidemic and if we don't stop it, it is going to kill us and our children and shorten our lifespans.

Did you know that diabetes is more than just your glycemic index, A1C or your insulin production? You don't just adjust your diet, watch your weight and go out jogging and you'll be fine. You have to watch how many restful hours of sleep you're getting. Yes, research has stressed time and time again the powerful connection between sleep and diabetes as well as other medical illnesses.

Have you seen very much on sleep as it relates to diabetes and obesity anywhere? I don't think you do because there's not enough of a corporate push behind sleep as there is behind the food industry, the pharmaceutical dietary supplement industry and the diet industry. Then, of course, there's also the exercise and fitness industry. *None of them mention sleep once.*

Why do you suppose that show "The Biggest Loser" was popular? Yes, perhaps there's also the exercise industry with its latest twist on sweating those calories away and developing that lean muscle that will make you someone who gets more than a second look by passersby. But, again, who's addressing sleep as a MAJOR component in diabetes and insulin resistance?

## Sleep medications, dementia and side effects

Sleep medications are sometimes prescribed, on a short-term basis, for certain times when insomnia caused by personal problems such as death of a loved one or a job loss or financial losses. But, overall, most healthcare professionals do not suggest they be taken regularly, even for those who have a nightshift job and may find it difficult to sleep during the daytime.

Until April 2019, the boxes for these medications contained the usual information on usage and contraindications but a study of adverse events by the US Food and Drug Administration revealed troubling statistics. The result was the "black box" warning. Any person who had had prior episodes of sleep disturbances, such as sleepwalking, were advised that these medications might be contraindicated.

The most popularly prescribed medications, i.e., eszopiclone (*Lunesta*), zaleplon (*Sonata*) and zolpidem (*Ambien, Ambien CR, Edluar, Intermezzo and Zolpimist*), were checked for adverse events in patients using these medications. The side effects appeared to occur whether the individual took only one dose or after longer periods of treatment and they were sobering.

*Sixty-six cases* were found to have resulted in serious injury or death after using eszopiclone, zaleplon or zolpidem. Patients experienced sleepwalking or driving, and 46 cases of nonfatal serious injuries were also noted. Of these cases, there were incidents of accidental overdose, falls, burns, near-drowning, exposure to extreme cold temperatures leading to limb loss or near death, self-injuries from gunshot wounds and suicide attempts.

*Twenty deaths* by patients on these medications were precipitated by carbon monoxide poisoning, drowning, fatal falls, hypothermia, fatal motor vehicle crashes with the medicated patient driving and seeming suicide.

Although the regulatory authority considered these cases "rare," they believed that the warnings needed to be placed on the boxes. When we consider that the US Centers for Disease Control and Prevention (CDC) has estimated that between *50-70 million* people in the United States take these medications, it becomes a serious health issue which must be addressed through patient and physician advisories.

The medications can provide relief from insomnia, but they must, considering the potential for serious side effects, be taken cautiously. Additionally, alcohol may potentiate the effects of the drugs, meaning make them more powerful, a similarly dangerous side effect should someone consumes alcohol while using sleep pills.

Should anyone avoid sleep medications entirely? The question is best left for a doctor-patient discussion.

One additional concern with regard to sleep medications is whether or not they may be involved with dementia, although the mechanism of action may not be fully understood at this point in time. However, we do know that over-the-counter (OTC) sleep aids, specifically those with an antihistamine effect (such as Chlor-Trimeton), appear to be involved in dementia long after the patient stopped taking the OTC pills. Antihistamines are often taken to treat allergies but also have a sleep-inducing quality.

In a seven-year follow-up of patients in a study of almost 3,500 men and women over the age of 65, who did not have symptoms of dementia, the researchers found that nearly 800 developed dementia. The dosage for the OTC medication was 4mg/day for at least three years. Additionally, the researchers concluded that the higher the dosage of the OTC medication, the greater the risk for dementia. Therefore, taking OTC medications is not without risk of dementia.

## weight gain, sleep and jet lag

Weight gain, as was just explained in the prior paragraphs, can be directly related to disruption in sleep and changes in hormones in the brain that control appetite. Not only does sleep deprivation precipitate changes in appetite, it may have a specific effect on one aspect of our eating – junk food cravings.

The mechanism that is activated appears to be related to what is called the endocannabinoids which regulate appetite and, yes, they are the same receptors where marijuana is bound. Interesting that carbohydrates, sleep and marijuana share a few things in common.

Lack of sleep appears to cause an increase in a specific blood concentration of this endocannabinoid which then results in an increase in appetite. The food intake was carbohydrates, fats and proteins, but I suspect that carbos led the pack.

I have been in hospital settings where nursing staff have worked long shifts and sometimes double or triple shifts (during intense snowstorms). What did they have in their offices? There was a complete vertical file cabinet filled with carbohydrate-rich snack foods to which they made regular trips.

I also did original research on binge eating in women over the age of 30 in the 1990s. Most of the women in my study were nurses who worked in research hospital programs around the United States.

Once the materials were in and the results were calculated, we found that just about 80% of the nurses were binge eating at some point and age wasn't a factor. The nurses did not, however, have eating disorders per se. Researchers today are now looking far beyond teens for binge eating since it appears in both males and females and at all ages.

# CHAPTER 11

# Sleep in medical settings

◆ ◆ ◆

*Sleep is when all the unsorted stuff comes flying out*
*as from a dustbin upset in a high wind. - William Golding*

Medical illnesses often result in sleep difficulties either because of pain in some instances or insomnia caused by as-yet unknown biological causes. Sleep, therefore, because of its restorative activities is essential and yet almost impossible for too many people.

Have you ever been a patient in an intensive care facility such as post-surgery where you were placed for a period of days in a unit where the lights never go out and the machines continuously make buzzing or whir-ring sounds and people are shuffling 24 hours a day? The level of intense stimulation can prevent sleep unless you are provided with sleep medica-tions and sometimes that's not in the medical protocol.

So, awake you stay while your senses are assaulted with all manner of sound, vibration and poking. Lack of sleep shouldn't be a given because you need your immune system and that brain cleaning to be working at optimum strength, but it's not. The ICU keeps buzzing along as it must and while staff try urgently to help those in distress, the rest of the patients lie awake and frightened.

How many times have we watched patients in these settings who begin to display bizarre behavior, attempting to escape or striking out at staff in the belief that they are there to hurt, not help, them? It is something called "intensive care syndrome" or psychosis and it's not uncommon especially in older adults.

I have seen ICU patients try to escape from a unit after pulling IV lines out of their arms and staggering down a hallway, leaving a telltale trail behind them. One man managed to make it past the nurses' station to the elevator in his hospital gown before I alerted staff that he was about to leave the floor.

The man in this instance was in obvious distress and mumbling incoherently as the nurses gently guided him back to his bed. It was fortunate that he was stopped in time.

## ICU syndrome

The symptoms that appear in the ICU can be misdiagnosed, especially in the elderly, as I said, as signs of dementia or a psychiatric disorder. Unless there's adequate attention to the stimulus overload leading to lack of sleep, the result may be inappropriate medications. What they are actually experiencing is a form of psychosis where normal reality testing is distorted into fearsome situations. Sometimes the most obvious cause of the mental impairments is right under their noses, but they don't see it.

When a patient is hearing impaired, as many elderly can be, the situation becomes even more dire. If these patients become agitated or, as in the case of a deaf individual, use their hands in ways not understood by staff, the use of restraints only exacerbates a bad situation to a worse one.

If you have an elderly person in your care and they undergo hospital-based medical procedures that involve an ICU stay, keep sleep deprivation in mind and advocate for conservative measures before anything more aggressive, such as antipsychotic meds, is brought to bear. Some psychotropic meds, if given to elderly patients, can cause death and are counterproductive, but staff may not have sufficient experience or knowledge in gerontology.

## Psychotic symptoms

Too often the elderly are seen as manifesting psychiatric symptoms due to bias when the actual cause of their symptoms may be lack of sleep, diet, poor hydration, inappropriate medications or even loneliness. And loneliness isn't a psychiatric disorder, but a consequence of social isolation and an ICU is one of the loneliest places. Too much must be performed by too few staff in too little time with churning shifts of often tired trainees or caregivers. Read up on ICU psychosis because I think all of us need to be knowledgeable about it.

## Noise in the hospital

Have you ever been in a hospital and had to spend at least one night in an ICU or CCU? What was the one thing that interrupted your sleep most? Yes, they came by frequently to take blood pressure readings or check your vital signs, but what else? There's no quiet time. The lights are bright or dimmed a bit but there always noise, people moving about, banging equipment and talking. It's highly disruptive.

## Finding a sleep center

The need for sleep and the research that is drawing in more medical staff and medical facilities has been a boon for anyone who needs a sleep assessment. You may feel a bit at a loss if you believe you do need an assessment but there's no need to worry. You can get a listing of sleep centers wherever you live in the United States.

Several thousand accredited sleep centers now exist in many hospitals and free-standing sleep centers and sleep labs in the diagnostic services they provide. In fact, major hospital facilities will fold their sleep medicine service component into their pulmonary medicine specialization. This makes sense because sleep disorders may be a function of a breathing problem that needs to be addressed by a pulmonologist.

Of course, these assessments are costly as you well know, but in many cases, they may be covered by insurance or the hospital may have what is known as "charity care" available or might be willing to provide the assessment as part of a grant-funded research project. Consider all of the possibilities before you decide how you will be paying for it and don't be afraid to mention cost to them.

All of the sleep centers that are listed in the information that I have provided are accredited and manned by professionals with expertise in sleep medicine. One thing every patient needs to keep in mind is that you will want someone who is licensed, accredited and has special expertise. I mention this because there may be people who are offering you these services but who do not have the requisite background to provide the full array of assessments.

Sleep centers have become a part of most medical facilities worldwide but may not be listed in the usual resources found online. Unfortunately, the current ones may include only those located in the United States. Persons in other countries, however, will have other means to find a sleep center near them but it may take a bit of research. In the United States, using Google, go to this website: http://www.sleepeducation.org/find-a-facility. Here you can do a search to find a center within 5 to 100 miles of your location.

Should you have some question regarding whether or not the medical professional you are seeing for your sleep difficulties is certified, there is a website where you can check the names of all of those who are diplomates in sleep medicine.

Here it is the US verification site: Verification of Diplomates of the American Board of Sleep Medicine (http://www.absm.org/listing.aspx). Don't hesitate to contact them if you have any questions because any medical treatment or evaluation is too serious to be taken lightly or handled by someone who doesn't have the proper credentials.

# CHAPTER 12

# Sleep and work

◆ ◆ ◆

*I put a piece of paper under my pillow,*
*and when I could not sleep*
*I wrote in the dark. - Henry David Thoreau*

Work, to a great extent, is the way we perceive ourselves and it is the way we are perceived by others, too. It stands to reason, therefore, that we want to do our very best while working in order to bolster our self-esteem. We also want the respect from others for doing a good or better-than-good job. Sounds reasonable, right?

What can we do, other than keeping up with technology or our job requirements, to keep ourselves performing at our best? One way is to ensure that we get the sleep we need because work depends on it. There is no question that sleep is one thing on which we must not fool ourselves into thinking we can skip and still do well; we can't. But the demands of our 24/7 work world, made possible by virtue of the internet, is playing havoc with our work and our sleep schedules. The results, coming in yearly, are not promising unless we make changes both in our lives and in the corporate attitude toward sleep and its relationship to work.

## A worldwide phenomenon

The rush of competition around the world has resulted in unsettling work conditions for many countries where ramped up work requirements result in stress-related illness and death, in some cases. Writing in the *Japan Times*, Dr. Cesar G Lila dissected how Japan has been affected by the new work environment.

*"In Japan the number of cases submitted for compensation has increased significantly in the past few years. So, has the number of court cases in which the government refuses to compensate the victims' families. In Japan, if karoshi is considered a cause of death, surviving family members may receive compensation from the government and up to $1 million from the company in damages…"*

The grueling work schedule expected of employees in Japanese companies has resulted in a growing body of evidence that workers in many high demand industries suffer from low social support and increased risk of developing disease which includes myocardial infarction and stroke. It is believed that stressful work conditions are a component of this phenomenon.

If a young female trainee (Huang & Stapczynski, 2016) in an advertising agency, who was expected to work 65 hours of overtime a month, jumps out the window of her office building because she can't handle the hours required, do we hear about it? Before she died, she worked more than 105 hours of overtime in one month. And she's not alone. Read about the working conditions and suicide rates in factories in China.

Japanese workers, according to one source, sleep less than any other workers around the world. Lack of sleep has been recognized, in a quite unusual way, by the corporations. They have instituted what is known as "sleeping while present" and there is even a Japanese word for it, "*inemun.*"

In other words, naps have been included in their time at work. The problem is that employees may take these 15-minute naps, but they must remain seated upright and not bend over their desk. The corporations don't want them to appear slovenly. Some companies do allow for a 30-minute nap and others actually have a room set aside for naps.

Similar problems related to work stress were found in China, South Korea, and Bangladesh. Women were at higher risk, according to an article and in a 15-year study conducted in Denmark. There the researchers found that the greater the work pressure, the higher the risk for heart disease among women under the age of 52.

While we consider, again, medicine where the sleep deprived intern/ resident is trying to struggle through an extremely long and demanding shift, what about the other, and equally important, personnel on the unit? And that is still true, even though the rules have purportedly changed, but what about the nurses who work as part of the medical team?

Do you even think of how they nurses are affected and what is expected of them during a long shift? Nurses are probably one of the most, if not the most, vital members of the medical team, so let's give them their due.

## Sleep and work effectiveness

A study of sleep in 2018 delved into the subject of the beliefs workers have regarding their effectiveness and how sleep may play a role.

Effectiveness and productivity at work or in other areas of our life is of prime interest to most of us. A sleep study in America that was conducted by the National Sleep Foundation in 2018 found that 65% of those sampled believed that getting adequate sleep was the means to being effective the next day.

Even though most people in the sample indicated that good sleep or quality sleep, was of utmost importance to them, only 10% of those said that sleep was more important than other areas in their lives. The contradiction here appears to be something with which the people in the sample decided they could live without questioning or without resolving the problem for themselves.

Sleep, therefore, remains important as they have indicated and yet they fail to prioritize it even though they say it is important. The question remains whether or not people say what they truly believe or what they believe the researchers would like to hear. Such a question is always on researchers minds whenever any research is conducted, and it must be on the reader's mind right now.

The study also found that 35% of those in the sample indicated that they were either extremely or highly effective in their daily lives and 65 9% said they were very effective. Interestingly, the ones who believed that they were most effective after a good night sleep were in the top income brackets. They had college degrees, which must be considered as an income status contribution, in some way, to their feeling satisfied with their lives. Accordingly, they may have been free from the financial stresses of those in lower income brackets.

The items of fitness, nutrition, and sleep were most important to those in the seniors' group while work was important for persons of Hispanic heritage, younger adults and men. Young people, specifically those who were single, indicated that the most important issue in their lives was their social life.

Results of this research have an interesting relationship with what we know about periods in people's lives. A highly regarded research study, which was done many years ago, found that a man's life was divided into discrete periods and each of these periods placed an emphasis on a certain aspect of life.

A book, entitled *The Seasons of a Man's Life* by Daniel Levinson, based on the results of this study, outlined what he felt were the important factors in the four phases of life. They included early adulthood when dreams of success and a future career are being formed, and socialization remained an important factor. If socialization is so important, then sleep takes a back-seat and what happens to the ability to be effective the next day?

Wait a minute, what about the early bird versus those night owls? Don't some of us do better in the morning and others do better at night? Why is that? Are some of us just lazy and can't get ourselves moving in the morning?

Okay, let's go back to the biology of sleep or, more appropriately, to our genetic-makeup. There is some new research that's indicating it's all written in that specific genetic code we've inherited, so it's not laziness at all. It may be out of our control entirely, but once we do determine which we might be, it would be helpful to adjust whatever we're doing to that internal script in our genes.

What's a night owl to do? Well, if it's really something that you can't seem to shake (and who can shake loose from the grip of our genes?), you might consider work that fits your internal schedule. Sometimes, that's not a bad idea because some jobs do pay a night differential and for other jobs, things are pretty quiet at night.

There are people who do very well at night and will actually thrive in the nighttime environment. But there are also those of us who will find the nighttime is our time for dreaming. It can be a struggle, especially if you are expected to maintain a work schedule that doesn't mesh with your body's physical demands.

Shiftworkers are all around us. They deliver the mail, drive the trucks, pilot planes, work on the steamships, fill the factory lobster shifts and so many other jobs that we don't even know about. Without shiftworkers and those who toil in the night, we would not be as safe as we are or as productive as a society.

Work and work situations have changed dramatically over the past century and even the past decade or two.

Companies no longer close businesses for evenings because business and all types of work activities can be completed in a variety of countries in any number of settings, home included. This shift has created a work world that is in direct opposition to what our bodies 24-hour clock (actually it's been found to be a 25-hour clock) can handle biologically.

The demands and the times the demands are made mean adjustments to a lifestyle, social as well as personal, and some adjustments may not be possible. For example, the work schedules of police personnel are in direct opposition to what our internal clocks are programmed for. You can't turn a person's shift backward on the clock rather than forward and expect a good adjustment, but that's how police work shifts have traditionally been laid out.

Our body's internal clock, as I mentioned, is regulated by the suprachiasmatic nucleus or nuclei (SCN), a structure just above the nerve connections for the two eyes in the front section of the brain. Yes, this seems like a truly involved process, but you needn't worry; there will be no test for comprehension after you read this book. But, please, make notes if you wish to remember something.

The small SCN structure is also believed to be involved in bird migration where light passes into the brain through a somewhat fragile bony protective plate. In humans, this internal clock is also biologically set to function in a certain manner, but it probably happens by the light passing through our eyes, hitting our retina and then passing the light signal on from there.

Working against that clock can be the problem here. And this isn't just conjecture on my part. Researchers are studying this because it is causing discord in our social network and our communities.

Recently, I spoke to a 20-year veteran of a major police force. He indicated that, within 10 years of retiring, many former officers will be dead. The reason? Their work schedules which are aimed in direct opposition to their bodies' internal clocks.

A circadian clock illustration from the Salk Institute for Biological (www.salk.edu) studies indicates approximate times when certain functions or activities are active in terms of body temperature, blood pressure, melatonin secretion (the sleep hormone) and highest level of alertness.

Along with these clearly noted activities is another that we need to discuss. The stress hormone, cortisol, that clearly has been found to stubbornly remain at a high level during the early hours of sleep. This higher level of cortisol contributes to or promotes insulin resistance which then can lead to obesity and diabetes, as I've noted previously.

Cortisol which is also higher under situations of stress is associated with multiple physical problems. The areas or disorders affected include anxiety, depression, digestive problems, heart disease, weight gain, memory and concentration impairment and a decrease in the efficiency of the immune system, leaving you at risk of disease.

Since sleep-deprived persons have a disruption in their cortisol levels, there is an attendant negative effect and suppression of the immune system. The close association, therefore, between job-related stress and sleep disorders has this additional, highly deleterious effect on the body. There is no cheating on sleep because to do so is cheating your health and your body's ability to maintain it.

## Drowsy drivers

There is no question in anyone's mind that driving while sleep deprived or drowsy can lead to fatal or near-fatal results for the driver and everyone in the car or on the road. Not only is the ability to respond quickly to changing road conditions impaired, but the actual visual perception may also be affected in bizarre ways.

Some drivers report seeing animals running across the road when what they really saw can be understood as a dark spot or shadow. We've all seen those water illusions on the road while driving in hot weather, so we are familiar how this can happen even to the fully awake driver.

Who might be driving while drowsy? When you consider that some cabdrivers or emergency personnel must work shifts 12 hours or more, is there any wonder that they would be drowsy while driving home? Their work places them at high risk of being in a serious driving situation just as alcohol would affect someone. In fact, it has been suggested that sleep-deprived drivers are, in a manner of speaking, driving drunk.

How many accidents have there been on major roadways where huge commuter buses that regularly ferry people from New York to Boston or Washington DC or Atlantic City have an incredible number of casualties after a crash? What about the driver of the executive limo bus that was carrying comedian *Tracy Morgan* that crashed on the New Jersey Turnpike in 2014? Or the train operators on railways where they crashed while rounding a curve or entering a station platform.

Morgan's comedy writer was killed and Morgan was left with severe injuries. The driver of a Walmart truck that struck the limo hadn't slept, according to reports, in 24 hours.

The AAA for Traffic Safety indicated how serious the question of drowsy drivers can be. "*A foundation study completed in November 2014 found the impact of having drowsy drivers on the road is considerable.*

"*Drowsy drivers are involved in an estimated 21% of fatal crashes, up from 16.5% from the previous 2010 study, as most drivers drift out of their lanes or off the road. Drivers themselves are often crash victims who die in single-car crashes.*"

To help place all of this in perspective, the National Center on Sleep Disorder has placed a chart on their website for your review. The link is: http://bitly.com/2mEvyPG.

Although their chart is primarily relative to auto accidents, it can be used to look at the physical aspects of jobs. On-the-job stress can result in what is known as adrenal fatigue. The adrenal glands are where the hormone cortisol is made, and the usual activity of cortisol is to help activate someone when there is a threat. Work can produce this type of mental threat for the body and the result is ultimately fatigue and a lower resistance to pathogens because of the overload on our adrenal glands.

An additional study in France, investigating the effects of drugs, alcohol and drowsy driving, concluded that the drowsy driver was just as much at risk of an accident as those who had drunk alcohol. As many others had suggested, the danger of a sleepy driver cannot be overlooked when considering traffic accidents.

## Airline pilots and flight crews

How many trips have you taken on a plane? You usually sit, I imagine, in the waiting area just outside the jetway and as the crew goes aboard, you notice they have luggage with them.

Cabin staff have the most luggage and the pilot and a co-pilot usually are just carrying a briefcase or some small piece of luggage. Do you ever wonder what their lives are like on the ground when they're not flying? Probably not.

But if you did begin a conversation with a flight crew member, probably well away from their place of work, you might be quite intrigued by how their lifestyles are affected by their flight schedules. Many of them are in one town for one night, and off the next day on a four-hour flight or more with one stop somewhere, possibly a hotel the airline has booked for them. But where do they actually live? Don't most of us have a stable place we call "home?"

I asked one stewardess what her flight plan was on that particular day. She told me she would be flying six hours to the West Coast, then on to Hawaii and back again. It sounded like something close to 12 hours just to go coast to coast and then another six or seven hours over the Pacific, or am I wrong? She said she loved it, but I can't imagine how it might be affecting her.

Did her work schedule contribute to the cancer she developed in her brain by way of depressing her immune system because of lack of restful sleep? No one knows for sure. She has had to have brain surgery with a bone removed and replaced several months later. The surgeon was quite surprised by the extent of the tumor in her head and the possibility of further damage.

During one operation, the surgeon commented afterward, he was not sure he could save her sight.

I should mention that, in addition to sleep deprivation, these crews are also exposed to high levels of radiation in the air as they fly as much as 35,000 feet from the earth. That would seem to be an important research project for someone to conduct in the future. In other words, what is the relationship between sleep deprivation and various forms of cancer in flight crews?

Crew members often share their "home" with several other crew members, and I doubt many of them actually have a place of their own. They aren't there long enough with their hectic flight schedules. Pets? I'll bet they don't have pets, either, unless they have a roommate who's there all the time and doesn't work for the airlines.

Working on an airline isn't the glamorous job people may think it is. It's hard work, lots of flying and little sleep time between flights. An interesting fact I recently learned might be something you hadn't heard about.

Do you know that the crew isn't paid for actual flying time until the plane's wheels are off the ground? Why do you suppose they want everyone on and off the plane so fast? It's their salary they're worried about.

Half of the pilots in a study admitted that they rarely or never have an opportunity to get adequate sleep. They were open in their responses and stated that at least 20% of them had committed a serious error while flying and sleepy. Only slightly less than 20% of train operators said they experience what they call a "near miss" in terms of an accident because of their sleep-related difficulties.

Although not readily discussed, some airlines have taken to giving their pilots time off, while in the cockpit and on a long-haul flight over an ocean, to take a nap. During this time, the co-pilot is in charge. If you knew pilots were falling asleep on long-haul flights, why not put something in place which would address this and attempt some remediation?

The British Airlines Pilots Association said that pilots were exhausted by their workload and one in three admitted to waking up on the flight deck and finding their co-pilot asleep, too. I can imagine what a scare that was.

Another group of pilots working for an airline in Asia noted that pilots regularly went to sleep while flying and, occasionally, had a stewardess take control of the plane. In one instance, the plane fell 5,000 feet because the non-pilot turned the autopilot off.

## Police/Fire department schedules

Do you know anyone who works as a police officer or fire person? What are some of the problems that are endemic in the personnel? You've heard of major stress in personnel and directly related problems in their personal life outside the work setting, but how many police officers suffer from some form of addiction or anger management? What is the incidence of divorce and family discord? The facts speak for themselves and some of the problems may be related to their work schedules.

The risk of having a traffic accident for firefighters is also quite high. One study in Boston uncovered some very disturbing facts about firefighters and accidents. "*Sixty-one percent of firefighters' on-duty fatalities were caused by heart attacks or motor vehicle crashes.*

"*Heart attacks are the leading cause of death in both career and volunteer firefighters. Motor vehicle crashes are the second leading cause of death in volunteer firefighters and ranked third among career firefighters.*" How much sleep do firefighters actually get? In the fire house, they must have that "third ear" to listen for the bell to sound that there's another fire.

Besides firefighters and police, which other group of people in vital professions might suffer sleep stress? The answer is probably too obvious to mention.

## Medical staff

Although times have indeed changed, physicians in training still undergo what is one of the most grueling work schedules imaginable and they are not only sleep deprived, they make life-and-death decisions hour-by-hour. Many teaching hospitals may have indicated a change in work schedules, but like truck drivers, it's not always what it seems.

The calculating of time on duty, hours off to sleep and return to work may not be sufficient to allow for sleep especially when that sleep can and is interrupted multiple times by calls regarding patient care. The matter is a dire one and it is estimated that about *400 physicians commit suicide* each year in the US because of stress/burnout.

So, it's not just the digital business world that I spoke about before where persons who are trying to attain higher positions sacrifice sleep. In addition to residents and interns, I've seen physicians, who were responsible for patient care on a unit, sleep through an entire treatment team meeting as the nurse took notes and handed a sheet around for signatures. Of course, no one ever mentioned to the physician that he should be remaining awake for these meetings. Doesn't that go without saying?

We ask ourselves how the situation might have changed, especially after you read the following report on the Libby Zion case. But there is still the question of sleep deprivation for physicians, whether in training or not.

Just how do medical staff "balance" those lengthy 28-hour days you ask and so did a physician in a recent article. Read what Karan (2017) had to say and what influenced him (Williams) when he read about a well-known physician.

Sleep and sleep deprivation remain a serious concern for all of us and change must be made or people may die. In fact, we know that is a definitely possibility.

## The Libby Zion case

Medical staff are sleep deprived not of their own accord but that of an out-of-date hospital staffing system which lauds training pain and sleep deprivation as an important rite of passage. Although medical centers have indicated they have remediated the system, one has to wonder if we are all still being treated by sleepy residents and inexperienced, sleepy interns (or should I say PGY-1 personnel?). You might want to ask for a name and their status on the staff.

BTW, for those of you not familiar with that PGY term, it stands for "Post Graduate Year" and it tells you a lot about how many years of experience that physician has had up to that point after medical school. Keep it in mind because it can be useful.

In the case of hospital care, it's not a misplaced decimal on a spread-sheet, but a med order that can prove deadly as was the famous case of this young woman. She was the daughter of a well-known New York City writer and she had been taken to a major, prestigious New York City teach-ing hospital some years ago; Columbia-Presbyterian.

Libby Zion was an 18-year-old Bennington College freshman who was in the throes of a mysterious ailment with a high fever and jerking bodily movements when she was taken to the hospital in 1984.

Agitated and difficult to work with medically, the staff reviewed her prior record and determined she must have been suffering from a mental disorder. The supervising physician, who never actually saw her, ordered physical restraints and a powerful antipsychotic medication for her. This was to be a fatal mistake.

While in the hospital during those first few hours, Zion's temperature rose to an incredible 107 degrees. She went into cardiac arrest and died after the staff's futile attempts to resuscitate her. Problems of medical over-sight, sleep deprivation and lack of proper evaluation/supervision all came up in the ensuing lawsuit, Zion v. New York Hospital.

The Manhattan district attorney initially considered murder charges against the physicians involved in Zion's care, but did not pursue that conceivable indictment. Then, too, it's possible that a charge of man-slaughter could have been lodged because, while Libby Zion died, the physicians attending to her did not intend for that to be the ultimate con-clusion of the case.

The final legal decision in the case was one of equal blame on the part of the hospital and Libby Zion herself for not revealing that she had previ-ously used cocaine. Considering the condition in which the young woman came into the hospital, how could it have been possible for her to tell them that she had used cocaine? Not reality-based to my mind.

Libby Zion had also been prescribed and used, on a daily basis, a psy-chotropic medication that was contraindicated by the medication given to her in the hospital, although the physicians didn't know of her use.

The cause of death was, however, not determined, although it was sus-pected to be _serotonin syndrome_. The syndrome is caused by the interaction of two medications, one she took herself and at least one that was administered at the hospital.

This high-profile case did bring about changes in graduate medical education procedures. Afterward, there was a strict reduction in work hours for residents. No longer would they work more than 80 hours per week and no more than 24 hours in a row. But did that really resolve the matter?

## Medical education changes

Today, the New York State Department of Health Code, Section 405 is known as the Libby Zion Law and it is the one which places restriction on work shifts for interns and residents. Libby Zion's father, in an Op-Ed piece in the New York Daily News in 1997 wrote an article entitled, "Hospitals Flout My Daughter's Law" which said in part:

*"... After it became clear to everybody, including a New York County grand jury, that Libby's death was caused by overworked and unsupervised interns and residents, the Libby Zion Law was passed. No more 36-hours shifts for interns and residents, from now on, attending physicians would be at the ready to supervise the young, inexperienced student-doctors. To accomplish these aims, $200 million a year was settled on our hospitals, which had been running slave-labor camps on the excuse they couldn't afford to work interns and residents for 'only' 80 hours a week went into effect in 1989.*

*"All that happened was that the hospitals use the money for everything but its purpose. Nothing has changed, except more raises for attending physicians, more perks for administrators. And we wouldn't know this were it not for Mark Green, the public advocate, and a great reporting job by Esther Fein in the Sunday Times. Interns and residents are still being forced to work crazy hours, more than 100 hours a week, and there's no supervision. The hospitals and the medical establishment flout the law with unspeakable arrogance and smugness."*

A careful retelling of the events of the night Libby Zion was taken to the hospital can be found in the article "The Lasting Legacy of a Case That Was 'Lost" by Stephen Cohen in Penn State Law Review, 2014.

After reviewing the working conditions and medical settings outlined in the articles on the death of Libby Zion, you must ask yourself about the working conditions of people in other professions such as law, finance, and computers where excessive hours are expected. We do not know how many people will die from the ravages of sleep deprivation or the attendant physical ailments it will bring on. We also don't know the danger they place us in because they lose their ability to attend to a task such as keeping the national electronic grid safe, or our dams running properly or controlling the traffic in the skies.

## Nursing staff

In a blog on the website of the American Nurses Association it was noted that, "*according to ANAS 2011 Health and Safety Survey, about one in 10 nurses surveyed were involved in an automobile accident that they believe was related to fatigue from shiftwork. Moving forward, nurses must take action to protect themselves and others from the danger of drowsy driving.*" Therefore, just in this one study alone, 10% of the nurses were involved in auto accidents related to shiftwork.

The National Institute for Occupational Safety and Health has found the situation sufficiently serious to issue a module for training nurses on shiftwork difficulties and possible routes to remediation regarding sleepiness. They also included a short video with additional work-related resources on their website for shift workers.

Additionally, there is an online training courses for nurses and their managers. Medical staff often have to catch a bit of sleep as they can with frequent awakenings through any rest they may have. How does that affect their quality of sleep? I think you know the answer to that one because there's little opportunity for sleep in these jobs.

One additional fact needs to be mentioned as it concerns nurses. The suicide rate of nurses is rising and must be addressed, as has been mentioned by the major suicide-prevention groups and hotlines. Along with suicide of physicians, nurse suicides remain hidden for the most part but must be addressed.

## EMS workers

Anyone who is either a volunteer or an employee of an Emergency Medical Service (EMS) understands that it's sleep while you can and be ever on the alert for that call. The call may be a matter of life or death and we have to wonder how maintaining such high alert would have prompted Dr. Hans Selye to comment on it if he were around to do that. Of course, he wasn't studying EMS personnel when he came up with his theory of how stress works and the steps involved in it, but it does fit into the EMS worker's life.

## General Adaptation Syndrome

Selye was responsible for what is known as the General Adaptation Syndrome (GAS) theory of stress. The characteristics, which were outlined by Hans Selye had three specific stages:

### *Alarm*

The brain receives a message indicating danger and begins to send out a signal for the release of cortisol and adrenaline to increase heart rate and energy with a resulting rise in blood pressure. Glucose in the blood also rises. This is the beginning of the "fight or flight" response.

### *Resistance*

The body attempts to return all system to a more normal level of functioning, but if the threat persists, this will not occur. Concentration is inhibited and irritability begins to show.

### *Exhaustion*

If the stress still persists for a *prolonged period*, the body progresses into this final, and most deadly phase, of the syndrome. The body's energy resources have been depleted and the result may be a feeling of tiredness, depression, anxiety, a sense of not being able to cope any longer, and health-related disorders may develop. Animal studies have shown this phase can mean the death of the animal.

## Tips for shift-workers and others

Government agencies have provided a number of sleep tips for shiftworkers, but primarily these are tips that are more useful for the regular daytime worker. Often, shiftworkers are working at night and trying to sleep during the day. Sometimes it's impossible for them to switch their shift around and that causes additional problems with their circadian or sleep clock.

The National Sleep Foundation suggests that in order to stay alert on your shiftwork job that you do the following:

Avoid long commutes and extended hours

Take a short nap breaks throughout the shift, if possible

Work with others to help keep you alert

Try to be active during breaks (take a walk, shoot hoops in the parking lot or even do a bit of mild exercise)

Drink caffeinated beverages to help maintain alertness during your shift

Don't leave the most tedious or boring tasks to the end of your shift. Night shift workers are most sleepy between 4-6 AM

Ask colleagues what they do to cope with the problems of shift work

## Tips for sleeping during the day

Wear dark glasses to blot out the sunlight on your way home

Keep to the same bed time and wake time schedule, even on weekends

Eliminate noise and light from your sleep environment (use a sleep mask or earplugs)

Avoid caffeinated beverages and food close to bedtime

Avoid alcohol because, although initially it may help improve sleep, tolerance develops quickly, and it will soon begin to disturb your sleep. In addition, alcohol can bring on depression because of its effect on the brain.

## What do actual shiftworkers do?

Following the guidelines of the NSF may not really fit for you, so we looked at suggestions from actual shiftworkers to see how they managed to cope in the world that is other than 9 – 5. Here's what they said helped them:

A nurse at a hospital who has a 7 PM – 7 AM shift three nights a week indicated that her biggest challenge is her social activities. She said that on her first day or night off she spends a few hours just taking it easy. What does she call it? It's her "nightshift hangover."

This nurse tries to group her shifts together so that she does have some consistency during the week and tries to exercise before going into work and to get out into the daylight, if possible. Naps are a regular part of her schedule, if she can fit them in.

A TV producer has to cope with the schedule that flips back and forth. One week he's on a 9 – 5 schedules, then the next week he has a night schedule of 5 PM – 1:30 or 2:30 a.m. Every other week, he rotates back again. Although it might seem hectic to most of us, he finds there are advantages such as going shopping, to the bank, keeping doctors' appointments but evening school activities with his kids really don't fit into his schedule. He's tired most of the time and he tries to take a nap, but he has little children at home and that's difficult.

A fellow who works in TV commercials finds that his work often goes from 4 AM to 4 PM, many times without notice. For him, days are often 12-hour stretches at a minimum. The schedule presents many problems since he is married and has home responsibilities and he finds that his sleep loss is very difficult for him.

The typical schedule of shooting a commercial often means that he has a total of 8.5 hours to shower, sleep, get up and make the drive back to work. Because of the nature of the work and the unpredictability of when work will come, he suffers with an excessive amount of anxiety and avoids making any commitments for social plans with family or friends.

The best thing for him, he states, is sleep. He and his wife have little time together because when he comes home he has to help sort out the bills, walk the dog and check the email. Blackout curtains in the bedroom are a must.

A fire lieutenant has a schedule where he's 24 hours on and then 48 hours off. Again, sleep is an extremely difficult commodity for him and he often finds that he only gets three hours on his shift days and sleeps at odd times on his days off. Often, his sleep is broken into blocks of time when he gets a few hours around noon and then a few hours around 11 PM. Doesn't sound like he ever gets seven hours straight.

From just these few illustrations, it is quite apparent that shiftworkers do not have an easy life, nor are they able to get the seven hours that is usually recommended for most people in terms of sleep. We can only suspect that shiftworkers are tired, sleepy and even may have impaired concentration. How can anyone work that way? Of course, there may be schedules that do allow for a decent, lengthy restful sleep, but too many shift jobs are not fashioned in that manner. It's inhumane in my opinion.

# CHAPTER 13

# Sleep in Space and Naps

◆ ◆ ◆

*It's easy to sleep floating around - it's very comfortable*
*But you have to be careful*
*that you don't float into somebody or something! - Sally Ride*

The whole question of whether space explorers could sleep in space has been largely settled by the information gleaned from the many missions initiated by NASA, the Russian Federal Space Agency, the European Space Agency, the China National Space Administration, the Japan Aerospace Exploration Agency and the Indian Space Research Organization.

The conclusion of all these organizations is that sleep is possible, but there are differences in terms of restfulness and the length of time for sleep space travelers can remain in the sack. The new normal of space appears to be about six hours, somewhat shorter than optimal here on earth. Agencies are quite conversant with the attendant difficulties of prolonged physical and mental effort and this brings sleep into clear focus.

How will space workers function under the shorter sleep spans, will they retain the sharp cognitive abilities and focus for the many demands of space travel? What will the long-term consequences of space travel be on the human body and will there be permanent or transient changes with which to contend?

How will mental health be affected? We've already seen that prolonged space travel can affect someone's genes as has been shown by the recent space trip of 340 days of Scott Kelly. Kelly came back with genetic changes and is now different from his identical twin.

Sleep aids, most probably because of side effects and considerations of chronic administration, would not be reasonable for space travel. However, a solution is currently being worked on that would also be helpful in certain operating room situations here on earth.

It's called cryogenic sleep and the mechanism is to place the person in a medically-induced sleep for prolonged periods in the OR and also to increase survival rates in persons with gunshot wounds. Whoever thought that procedures in the operating room could be translated to space travel?

Anyone who is a fan of the TV director/writer, Rod Serling, will appreciate this consideration. Ever see the *Twilight Zone* episode with William Shatner where he is in a plane and sees a creature on the wing? You can catch it on YouTube if you do a n internet search.

## Space and the space-sleep frontier

Is Shatner mad or is there really something out there? Think of the scenes in "*2001 A Space Odyssey*" where the travelers are placed in suspended animation chambers to be put to sleep for the months, perhaps years-long journeys into outer space.

When we first saw this, it was science-fiction. Today, it may be closer to reality than we think because NASA has been studying this possible prolonged sleep state for years. But the astronauts will wake up older and how will their muscles work, their reflexes, their minds?

Space and our wish to explore the enormity of the universe as we know it and discover universes yet to be seen means that sleep will enter a new phase of research. This research will take place in atmospheres far different from anything we have encountered on earth. The grand new adventures have, even now, begun a quest in sleep research laboratories bent on providing new insights thanks to new environmental factors.

Each move into these artificial atmospheres where day and night are no longer governed by the rising of the sun and setting of the moon may uncover scientific gold. Those who make the initial discoveries will undoubtedly reap the benefits in terms of career and professional profile advancement. But there will also be suffering.

We're humans on earth, but what about those who venture into space? What effect will it have on sleep?

Suspended animation where astronauts are placed into a state of prolonged sleep may solve the many difficulties of sending them on missions where it will take 180 days to reach Mars. The logistical problems? How about providing enough food, water, energy and even meaningful activity? Huge amounts of provisions would be needed and that would weigh down the craft, slow it down and make it prohibitively expensive. Sleep, therefore, may come to the rescue of space travel.

A recent discovery of astronauts in terms of their health after periods in space is that their brains float higher in their heads. Not only that, but space travel can change one's DNA as was found in the experiment of the twin American astronauts, Mark and Scott Kelly. While one remained on earth, his brother stayed in the international space station for one year.

Upon returning to Earth, the researchers found that Scott had a change in his genetic expression which they found insignificant. The changes were related to immune system, DNA repair, and bone formation networks. But he also showed slower cognition on tasks on Earth and there may have been other, not noticed now, that will erupt at some time in the future.

## What will happen to sleep in space?

Space travelers will not just voluntarily go to sleep because no one can sleep for months on end and that goes without saying. How many of us can sleep 9 or 10 hours unless we just worked 24 hours straight? Our bodies rebel against excessive sleep it seems even if we'd like to force it to get more hours of sleep.

One study of 64 astronauts who traveled on 80 space shuttle missions and another of 24 astronauts who worked on the International Space Station, found that they slept six hours a night on average. This was a change from their usual schedule which called for 8.5 hours of sleep.

The future efforts regarding how space travel or sleep while in orbit will affect astronauts will need to look at a number of behavioral health and performance issues. These include workload, sensory stimulation and stresses. Some of the changes which have been under consideration regarding the physical layout of the space station include changes in the types of light bulbs that would be used in order to have less of an effect on the astronauts' circadian rhythms,

One of the most prevalent findings of astronauts was that they complained of sleep deprivation and fatigue. Because of the lack of gravity in space flight, astronauts generally are either strapped in place to prevent them from floating around or they sleep in small container-like areas which must be adequately ventilated to prevent carbon dioxide from accumulating around their head. They also need to dim instrument lights and ensure that there is adequate sound proofing of any type of pump in the cabin.

Generally, astronauts work 10-hour workdays for three days a week and this can be more than 60 hours per week. Such a high-intensity workload does result in physical and mental fatigue which can have critical effect on cognitive performance and even in self-evaluation of their performance. Fatigue, therefore, in terms of inadequate sleep, is of primary concern in space travel.

The influences that were most noted to be problematic while in space included noise, physical discomfort, disturbances caused by other crew-members and temperature. Factors that were involved in changes which were problematic, in terms of astronauts' circadian rhythm, included shift work, extended work hours, timeline changes, sleep shifting, prolonged light of the lunar day, and abnormal environmental cues such as unnatural light exposure.

### *Melatonin capsules and sleep pills*

Sleeping pills are not the answer, either, but some astronauts did need to use them in space. But even over-the-counter preparations may have undesirable side effects and some of them, such as melatonin, may not have the total dosage indicated or have other, unlisted, ingredients (Erland, 2017). There is little, if any, regulation on some of these products and you should remain aware of this as you shop. No, you're not a space traveler but a wise consumer.

Melatonin was indicated to have an effect on circadian rhythms in persons with autism (Ann, 2016) and it is, therefore, advisable to proceed cautiously. If you explore some of the highly disturbing side effects and the lawsuits around the sleep aids and the consequences of using them chronically, you may be amazed. Try doing a search on the Internet for any of the following:

Barbiturate
Benzodiazepines
Bromide
Hypnotic
Nightcap
Sedatives-hypnotic
Sedative
Sleep aids
Sleeping tablet
Soporific

Of course, you can Google (or Duckduckgo if you prefer another US search engine) the brand names of some of the sleep aids with which you are familiar or go to the Physicians' Desk Reference (PDR) found in any reference section of your local library. There's also *The Peoples' Pharmacy* online. There you can find the listing of the side effects (some more usual than others which are seen as rare) or AEs (adverse events) as they're known in the medical world.

How are medication side effects rated as "not unusual" and how is one seen as "rare?" You might think that there's some special formula to come up with this system of ratings, but there actually isn't a rating system but a reporting activity. It's all a matter of the individual researchers involved in the clinical trials who have reported what they'd seen or have chosen to not report. And it also depends on the ethics of the person reporting.

I recall a clinical trial of a medication for a neurologic disorder where one woman developed a rash. Rashes are warning signs of possibly a very serious medical condition such as <u>Stevens-Johnson Syndrome</u>, a somewhat rare, life-threatening skin condition seen in some persons allergic to a medication.

The woman in question had suddenly developed the rash after taking the study medication. The cautious, and to be congratulated, physician reported the AE to the pharmaceutical firm running the study.

What the person caring for the elderly woman forgot to consider was that the woman had used a new skin cream the day before and it was the cause of the rash. However, rash was included in the PDR record for the med when it was finally marketed because, once reported, the AE must be included as a precautionary measure.

CHAPTER 14

# Sleep & creative dreaming

◆ ◆ ◆

*Mother believed that I should have an enormous amount of sleep,*
*and so I was never really tired when I went to bed.*
*This was the best time of day,*
*when I could lie in the vague twilight, drifting off to sleep,*
*making up dreams inside my head the way they should go. - Sylvia Plath*

After all the information about why you need to sleep, what happens if you don't sleep and the disorders, both physical and mental, how about some more *positive information on sleep*? For example, what about dreaming and its relationship to creativity or problem-solving or enhancing self-esteem, or consolidation of memory, or growing new sprouts in your brain for new connections? All sound good, don't they? Yes, of course they do, and you benefit from the use of a lot of them as you sleep.

You may still feel guilty about getting enough sleep because you "feel" you shouldn't and that it's a waste of time and you need to be productive. Hogwash. Don't buy the urban myth that sleep is a waste of time because now you know definitively, that it is not. Sleep is time well spent and it will enhance and, possibly, prolong your life, your health, your career and your lifestyle.

Sleep can relieve stress, get those wonderful little cleaners busy with their mops and brushes in your brain and help maintain all the internal plumbing in the process. Speaking about plumbing, remember that sleep and kidney connection? Well, no one wants to be hooked up to a dialysis machine for hours on end, so sleep and keep that thought in mind that you are warding off such unwelcomed interventions.

Anyone who ridicules sleep is uninformed but if they want to spend their time in physicians' offices or taking a handful of pills, it's their choice. You don't have to proselytize about sleep, and you don't have to stand up on a soapbox in the office and shout out sleep's values, either. Just stick quietly to your routine and enjoy your life.

Think of it as your creative self that is switching into high gear as your brain goes about the business of preparing for the next day. The brain truly is one of the most amazing parts of your body and has potential for many different types of activity during sleep that I don't believe have yet been tapped. It's still holding out on us.

There are more secrets to be discovered, but perhaps, if we'll listen to a few people relating their really interesting sleep and dreaming experiences, you can begin to work on your new sleep time efforts, too. Who knows, you might get a great idea for a book, a career or even a computer program and it's just a matter of getting a bit of shut eye. Sleep may be the truly creative key to certain types of success.

## Stephen King, author

Stephen King is probably, outside of Joyce Carol Oates (who is a marathon writer), one of the most successful, dedicated and hard-working writers on the American scene today. His work is quickly devoured by his increasing numbers of fans and King, I have to say, is a very fine writer. Just pick up anything he's written and see for yourself because it is a real treat.

Whether you like fiction that is somewhat scary or not, you can't deny the perfection of one of King's tales. But King has admitted that he has used something called "creative sleep." King isn't actually asleep because he indicates this part of his creative process happens even when he's in a wakeful dream state prior to a deep sleep. The incredibly successful writer has offered some practical tips to anyone who wishes to try their hand at being more creative and utilizing this wakeful dreaming.

What he recommends, and this is very similar to what we have talked about in terms of sleep hygiene, is that you place yourself in a room that only needs to have one thing; a door that you are willing to shut. As he indicates, when that door is shut it's your time to tell the world that you are at work.

King recommends no distractions in that room, including no telephone, no TV, no video games and if there is a window, you should pull down the shade. I think this would work also for creative daydreaming, something I find very helpful when conceptualizing something like a design, a book or any project.

This latter suggestion by King reminds me of what Isaac Asimov once told me about his writing apartment in his Manhattan hotel suite. He chose the apartment because it had no view and the windows on one side of it looked out on a brick wall. This, he said, made sure there would be no distractions.

Actually, one of Stephen King's most popular books, which was made into a film, Misery, is the product of a dream that King had while he was on an airplane. The dream was a lot more gruesome than he portrayed in the finished novel and film. But the dream did provide the essential material that he worked into the plot.

In fact, King is quoted as saying, *"but I wrote the first 40 or 50 pages right on the landing here, between the ground floor and the first floor of the hotel."* I'd say that's pretty good writing speed for anyone, and I can't imagine how he got all of that down either on paper or in his mind. Extraordinary.

King isn't the only one who utilized a dream for a creative endeavor. You don't have to be a writer, but I suppose they can benefit most from it. Scientists, too, have found that dreams often provide clues to questions they strived to answer while awake.

## James Cameron on and The Terminator

The man who made the film, Titanic, isn't just a filmmaker, he's a qualified engineer, inventor, an ocean explorer who also happens to be a multi-mil-lionaire who owns an island off New Zealand. An incredibly accomplished filmmaker, one of his films, *The Terminator*, is the product of a dream or delusional state that Cameron had experienced during the time that he was sick with a fever of 102 degrees.

He admits that he had a "vision" of a robot in his room that was coming at him with a knife. Cameron was sleeping at the time, so obviously, it was a dream that he then utilized in writing his screenplay. Not only did he use this theme in writing the screenplay for that film, but it also came in handy for his creative efforts on Avatar. Creativity is where you find it and for Cameron, it would seem, it lay in delusions during illness thanks to a fever.

## Mary Shelley on Frankenstein

How Mary Shelley came to write her classic novel, *Frankenstein*, is in itself an interesting story. Mary and her husband along with Lord Byron were spending a vacation in the Swiss Alps but a snowstorm trapped them in their lodge.

In order to pass time, they decided to have a writing competition with each one writing some piece of literature. Neither a theme nor any material seemed to come easily to Mary Shelley that evening, but little did she know that it was just waiting for her to go to sleep.

After she went to sleep, she recalled the next day that she had a "waking dream" that contained a monster and some very disturbing actions. Mary was quick to notice that, if she were feeling heightened emotion about the nature of the story, it would definitely have public appeal. She wrote the story about a misunderstood, ugly and frightening creature and the rest is history.

## Jack Nicklaus' golf swing

Do you engage in any type of sport and is there something where you'd like to improve your ability in that sport? Take a note from a champion.

Everyone who has any knowledge of golf, knows about the Golden Bear, who is more properly known as Jack Nicklaus, one of the most successful professional golfers in the game who is now retired. In golf, as in any sport, there can be difficulties with your skill in specific areas and Nicholas was no exception.

After a series of disappointing rounds of golf, Nicholas knew there was something wrong with his swing but he couldn't figure out what it was. In a dream, he saw himself addressing the ball with his golf club and notice that his grip was different. When he got up the next morning, he gave the grip that he saw in the dream a try and sure enough, it worked. He didn't really like to admit it, but the answer came to him in a dream.

## Invention of the sewing machine

Who would've thought that the sewing machine would be the product of the dream where Elias Howe had been given an order by the King to invent such a machine? In real life, Howe had been struggling with exactly how he could manipulate the needle to work in his new sewing machine invention. It was an extreme frustration for him.

At night, while he slept, he dreamed of that king who demanding the sewing machine be invented and, if he didn't respond to the king's demands, he was to be executed the next morning. The dilemma and the drama were there.

In the dream, the next morning came and Howe still didn't know what to do. As they marched him out onto the field to be executed, he noticed that the tips of the spears the soldiers were carrying were pierced. Suddenly, he awakened, went to his workshop and fashion the first sewing machine needle with a pierced tip. The dream had provided the design.

There are many other examples where dreams have helped people solve problems whose answers eluded them during their waking hours. Included in these examples are the understanding of benzene rings, the DNA molecule structure, even the periodic table used in chemistry. So, the mind is actively working on problems and problem solving as we sleep, but we may not even be aware of it.

Some people have espoused the idea that, if we have a particular project that is stymieing us, we sleep on it and allow our brain to do a bit of its own homework for us. Others have suggested that we actually formulate our sleep scenario for ourselves before we go to sleep. I suppose we could call this a form of sleep-problem-solution priming. That, of course, is my creative concoction and I do claim ownership of it. If you wish to use it, please give appropriate credit to me in any of your discussions.

## Placebo sleep

How many times have you read that someone took what was supposed to be a medication and it was actually a sugar pill and they achieved the result they sought? All of us know about the "placebo" effect where our belief is the thing that makes the result come to be, is not the "medication" we thought it was but a fake. In fact, there's even something called the "nocebo" effect

What's the difference and what is "placebo sleep?" First, what is placebo sleep? As explained regarding sleep and the placebo effect (Draganich, 2014), it's again the person's perception of their sleep quality after they were given arbitrary information, not actual information derived from study instrumentation.

Yes, they wired the participants up so that they thought they were actually being monitored by equipment, but it wasn't attached to any metering device. In research, it's called a ruse and often thought, in some research, to be totally unethical.

Those who thought they slept better (even though this was a lie), did better on a test of recall than those who were told they didn't have such good sleep quality. In other words, they believed what they were told and acted as though they had been affected by the quality of their sleep. What you believe about your sleep quality, therefore, can have a dramatic effect on your functioning the next day.

But it's not only how well you function mentally, but physically as well because a similar experiment was carried out with hotel housekeepers (Crum & Langer, 2007) who were told that the work they did was actually beneficial for him. What happened there? They essentially improved on measures of health relative to their perceived "work exercise."

The nocebo effect (also known as "placebo's evil twin"), as you might imagine, is when a harmless intervention or "medication" is given to a subject and they exhibit the negative results (the adverse events or AEs) they were told might occur. Not very nice, right? No, it wasn't, but it does prove how powerful our minds can be in terms of helping us face whatever we must and pushing on through.

Remember that great line from the film *"Field of Dreams"* where he hears a voice saying, "If you build it, they will come?" Well, if you think it, it just might happen. Isn't that the advice they give to all just-starting entrepreneurs?

No failure, no success is also another way to look at it. Failure isn't failure but information you use to take a different tack to approach an obstacle, be that a person or a business opportunity or sleep. Here, we're talking about sleep, so the ball's in your court, as I've said before.

## Using your night creativity

Each evening you are given a golden opportunity, whether you've ever thought about it or not, to utilize all of that brainpower that might not be used in cleaning up. It's not that the brain is lazy, it's just that it's waiting for you to decide how you might want to use it to best advantage for yourself. Don't let it just sit there. Use it!

If you have something that you might be able to work on as you sleep, go to it. Look at the examples that I provided about how incredibly successful people saw the opportunity that was presented in dream-like sequences that could be incorporated into their daytime activities. It's quite astonishing and you may be able to do some of it, too. Give it some thought and begin to keep a dream journal, not for therapy but for creativity.

Okay, let's look at a few things that you might be able to do tonight. Give yourself a chance to do a bit of experimenting. Never thought about yourself as an experimenter. Well, here's your chance.

You don't have to be an expert and you don't have to feel like you're going to be evaluated by anyone. After all, this is your workshop and you can use it as you wish. Take whatever you want, toss the rest aside, or begin anew. It's all up to you.

The pathway is being laid out for you each evening. See where it goes and take a look around at your own dreamscape. Can sleep actually have an effect on what or how you learn something? Let's see how it can be utilized to your best advantage and how sleep can have added benefits.

## Sleeping and learning

Sleep provides one of the best means of aiding you and your daytime memory. Of course, one of the reasons it can do this is because you allow it to process information that you've gone over just before you went to sleep. You can learn while you sleep (Anthony et al, 2012; Stromberg, 2012) because your brain is eager to do what we've been told to avoid; multi-tasking.

Whenever you have to remember some material, let's say you're trying to learn a computer program coding sequence or a language or something from a manual that you will need to use later or even prepare for a test, the time to go over it is *just before you go to sleep.*

An additional finding of sleep research may be something for the future in terms of learning. As we sleep, our brain's electrical activity goes through a series of waves. Some of these waves are referred to as spindles and this is where indications point to memory formation. A small study in the United States has shown that applying a tiny bit of electrical current via the scalp appears to enhance learning by augmenting the strength of these spindles. Exciting? Yes. Proven and workable right now? No, but something for future research.

Dreams may also be put to use, if you learn how to use the techniques, which aren't very complicated. Research that has gone on for over the past half-century points to your ability to utilize dream scenarios that you construct just before you go to sleep at night, too. What's your scenario to be? What do you want to accomplish for yourself the next day? What about for the next five years?

You can write a scenario where you are the main character and you can decide where you want to go and how you're going to do it. The purpose here is to help yourself improve your sense of self-esteem.

Don't give yourself anything too difficult, initially. Build up slowly with your nighttime scenarios and see how they work out during the day. Remember this is an experiment and all of it takes time, retooling and realization. If you want to play the violin in a concert, you first have to learn to play the violin. As the old joke goes, "How do you get to play at Carnegie Hall?" Practice.

One thing to remember, too, is that while you sleep and all those wonderful little biological cleaners are working, you are also relieved of the distractions in a normal day. Distraction during the day is one thing which interferes with learning but during sleep that is eliminated. This relief from distraction may be what is needed for memories to consolidate and new or stronger nerve connections to be formed. Freedom from distraction may well be the reason that learning before sleeping works so well.

Then, too, remember that reading in bed is a great way to help yourself get to sleep, so this learning/memory enhancement is an added bonus.

One additional interesting fact that has been discovered in sleep research deserves mention here. We know that coupling learning with something else can improve learning. For example, if you drink coffee or a particular type of soft drink or tea while studying some material, drinking that coffee later when *you're trying to recall* the material can actually help.

Studies have been completed in Europe by Ritter and her associates who used particular scents while people were learning a mathematical formula. During the night, while the persons in the research lab slept, the same scent was released into the room for some of the subjects but not for others. Those who were exposed to the scent as they slept remembered over 60 percent of the material where those who did not have the scent as they slept remembered less than one third of the material. It's believed that just the scent causes the brain to keep forming important new connections as the subject's slept.

You can certainly use this trick if you wish. If there is a particular scent you like, have it near you while you are studying any material or working on the creative project and then keep the scent near you where you sleep at night. See if it helps. If it does, you've just gotten a new way to help yourself with your memory and your creativity as you sleep. The process is amazing.

## Smartphone use

Smart phones do not direct our lives, nor should they be permitted to do so. Who does the permitting, anyway? We do. Therefore, it is within our purview to decide when and if these devices will be allowed in our lives.

As you've seen, the use of smart phones has contributed to problems in students and learning, levels of anxiety and mood disorders and general discomfort regarding our self-esteem and our place in our social sphere. What to do about this?

Researchers have several suggestions and I would think you will want to carefully consider each of them and see how *they might be helpful to you.*

Do you need to use your cell phone to list all your activities, to take notes, to maintain a calendar, and be your alarm clock?

Help yourself to stop checking your cell phone the first thing in the morning. It is not the most important thing in your life, unless you are an on-call ER physician.

Let people know that there are *certain times during the day and/or the evening* when you will not be available by cell phone or email. You do have a right to have dinner without interruptions or to engage in some other activity which is refreshing and which you enjoy.

Consider turning your cell phone off at night and even placing it in another room so that it's not readily available to interrupt your much-needed sleep.

When you are driving or trying to read and learn something, cell phone use should be eliminated or limited to very short periods of time and only as a true necessity. Interruptions are disruptions to your train of thought.

Checking your cell phone constantly or reading text messages constantly can only contribute to higher levels of stress and anxiety and do little, if anything, for you.

Wean yourself off this constant checking and remember that this is not going to be an easy task. Once you are so accustomed to this constant checking, it becomes a task where you really must apply yourself with diligence and stick to your resolve. That checking, too, is going to interfere with your best efforts to get a good night's sleep.

Technology is wonderful and extremely helpful, but we must still remain the ones in control. There is no reason to permit it to take over your life. But this can happen almost without our awareness. Take a few minutes out and consider it.

### Always remember this...

Always remember that sleep is a time for rest, even though your brain will be very active, as you know. A few simple techniques can help here, too.

Picture yourself lying on a cloud and easily settling into the softness of the cloud. Floating on it.

Tell yourself that now is the time for you to sleep and to relax.

Practice <u>deep muscle relaxation</u>. Relaxation can be helped along by beginning with your feet, then your legs, your stomach, chest and shoulders. With each part of your body, you allow the muscles there to completely relax. You probably don't realize how tense you are until you actively work to relax those muscles.

Drift off into the dream world you want to create and where you will find joy and fulfillment. You can work on the task you set for yourself anywhere you to daydream; on a beach, in a ski chalet, on a lake, in a garden swing, or walking in a field of sunflowers or a pine forest.

Sleep can be your most potent means of helping yourself to have a happier, healthier and more fulfilling life. Don't sell it short or let anyone badmouth sleep. It's the best medicine or therapy we have, and nothing will ever be what sleep can be for us. It's medicine, prevention and rejuvenation all rolled in one and there's no need to get anyone else to prescribe it.

# CHAPTER 15

# Some tips for you and employers

◆ ◆ ◆

*We are such stuff*
*As dreams are made on, and our little life*
*Is rounded with a sleep - Shakespeare*

Sleep requires a few simple things that all of us can do and it doesn't require spending any or very little money. Primarily, we have to concern ourselves with where we will sleep, how that space will be used and how to prepare it for optimal sleep production. It's not difficult and you will benefit from just a few simple changes.

What do we call this sleep-related effort on your part? *Sleep hygiene* and it is not centered around bathing, but rather *preparing your sleep space* for exactly that—sleep and nothing more.

Too many of us have become accustomed to using our bed or sleeping area for many purposes including working on our computers (remember that blue light?), making cell phone calls, watching TV or hanging out in that comfortable space we can call our own. But the experts on sleep medicine say that's where we're working against our sleep goals.

Your bed is not the place to do work, nor is it the place to play computer games or catch up on texting to family and friends. Both take away from that sleep you desperately want to catch up on in bed.

## Multi-step sleep hygiene checklist

Briefly, a review of some of the things which are included in what is known as "sleep hygiene," are listed here for easy reference. Let's take a look at some of the things you need to consider in your sleeping time and sleeping area so that you can optimize your sleep and utilize what science has provided for us in terms of sleep.

A simple *11-tips checklist* might be the simplest way to help yourself here, so let's take a look at the tips you need to follow:

Try to get up at the *same time each day.*
Go to bed only when you're going to go to sleep.

Establish what would be a relaxing pre--sleep routine for yourself such as taking a warm bath, having a light snack or doing a bit of meditation but *no vigorous exercise at least six hours before bedtime.*

Mild exercise, including simple stretching or walking, *at least four hours* prior to bedtime would be preferable, if that is something you find helpful.

Try to keep a regular schedule of activities. The schedule includes mealtime, when to take your medications, if any, what chores you do and at what time and on what days. Any other activities which, when kept on a regular scheduled basis, will enable your "body clock" to be kept running smoothly.

No caffeine after 12 PM.

No alcohol. Alcohol may make you feel tired at first, but it interferes with your ability to get restful sleep at night.

No tobacco because tobacco is a stimulant and will also interfere with your bedtime. It is interesting to note that there are nicotine receptors in the spinal cord.

If at all possible, and you find naps are helpful during the day, try to take them at the same time each day, usually *around the mid-afternoon* when your circadian rhythm is lowest, and limit the nap to about 20 minutes.

If you must use sleeping pills, use them only on an *occasional basis.* Sleep medication has been found to be both helpful and harmful if used chronically, a.k.a., each night. Too many reports of persons having abnormal, bizarre behavior while under the influence of sleep medications, improperly used, have been reported in the media.

Remember to *keep that sleep log* and make it a practice of putting something into it each evening. The notation should reflects what has happened during the day and, as you do an analysis, it may spark a sudden realization of what is interfering with your ability to sleep at night.

Be sure that your sleeping area is quiet and free from as much light as possible. Blackout curtains or shades are useful.

Keep your sleeping area cool.

## Alcohol use

Too often, alcohol is seen as a means of getting to sleep or improving sleep, especially in those who have chronic insomnia. Studies of persons who use alcohol as a sleep aid indicate that after three nights of alcohol use the initial sedative effect wears off and a tolerance develops. The tolerance can lead to improper use of alcohol which is non-therapeutic in nature and carries with it many more problems. It hormonal issues, especially those related to the nervous system and levels of anxiety.

Active daytime alcohol users, not just bedtime users of alcohol, who also have a sleep disturbance, number between 30-80% in terms of alcohol users who indicate they need alcohol for sleep. Sleep disruption then complicates their alcohol withdrawal since the tolerance that they have developed interferes with their alcohol rehabilitation. Unfortunately, too many people believe that this substance abuse is a soporific and they, in particular, are at increased risk for alcohol abuse.

Prior use of alcohol to induce sleep has led some persons to believe that it can be a harmless and effective means of returning to a restful night. For some nonalcoholic persons it may help, initially.

Chronic bedtime alcohol use increases what is known as *sleep latency*, or the amount of time from going into bed to actually going to sleep. These individuals, once they awaken the following day, will experience problems in learning, memory, and cognitive performance because alcohol suppresses an important sleep stage, REM sleep. REM is where information consolidation and memory formation are important brain activities.

As little as *one drink at bedtime* has been shown by research studies to lower restorative sleep. It is estimated that up to 30% of people who report persistent insomnia in the general population have indicated that they have used alcohol to help them get to sleep.

Sleep isn't the only issue where alcohol consumption, in terms of health, must be considered. Alcohol does possess what is known as a "feel good effect" but excessive drinking, as we know, brings with it a high risk of dementia. Even moderate drinking, defined as no more than one drink a day for women and two for men, has detrimental effects on the brain.

An extensive study of 10,000 people in Europe looked at their 30-year alcohol intake on memory tests and MRI scans. What they found was that there was shrinkage of the brain in the area, the hippocampus, associated with memory and reasoning and it was related to the amount of alcohol that the person drank.

Six times the risk of dementia of this type of drinking was found in persons who had at least four or more drinks a day. For those who had moderate drinking histories, their risk was still three times as high for brain impairment as those who were not drinkers.

Another study of almost 3,500 men and women found that brain shrinkage was greater even in persons who had light and moderate alcohol drinking histories when compared to people who didn't drink at all. An additional concern regarding breast cancer in women has been flagged as of interest and women who had one drink a day had an *increased risk of breast cancer* of 8.25% to 8.8%.

## Exercise

The question of exercise is one that is still being debated as a benefit or a hindrance to attaining the sleep that you need each evening. While sports in the evening, after work, may be enjoyable, some feel that it is too invigorating and leads to less restful sleep. However, others, to the contrary, believe that sleep is not affected if the vigorous exercise is limited to no more than one hour closer to your bedtime.

In other words, vigorous exercise is fine as long as you go to sleep at least an hour afterward. The "golden hour," therefore, is your determinant when looking at the time that exercise would be appropriate and the time when it wouldn't.

How do you determine what constitutes vigorous exercise? According to some experts, vigorous exercise leaves you unable to speak to another person during or just after it. Moderate exercise, on the other hand, can be signified by being able to speak to another. Such a standard would appear to be simple to follow.

But there are many other ways to gauge whether exercise is vigorous or not and that may be left up to the person completing the exercise routine. Judge for yourself and act accordingly.

## Forest bathing

Walking in the woods, or forest bathing as it's known, isn't just a pleasant activity because research has shown that not only does it provide a feeling of well-being, but it lowers the stress hormone, cortisol. Forest bathing also lowers your pulse rate and your blood pressure and seems to give your entire nervous system a much-needed break from the stresses of your life. Undoubtedly, it is something that should be considered in any plan to improve your life circumstances and your outlook.

Do you need a forest? No, you can enjoy forest bathing at a local park, a wooded area or anywhere there are trees and a sense of peace. I've been to an arboretum where there's an enormous and old Weeping Ash tree. The tree is so large that you can walk beneath it and there you'll find a wooden bench inviting you to come and sit for a while and enjoy the peaceful presence under the tree which almost embraces you. It is a very peaceful place and a calming experience.

Do you need any equipment to forest bath? Again, the answer is no. Your two feet will do nicely. Your only "equipment" is to select the place to pick for this activity. Once there, you can allow yourself the freedom of concentrating on the moment, push negative thoughts away, do some relaxation breathing and allow yourself a breather from stress.

Remember that the prime reason here is to allow you to lower your stress. Lowering stress will help you get that night's sleep you want and you will receive the benefits that sleep brings.

After reading about the benefits of forest bathing, perhaps a free starter kit might be what would be helpful. You can find one at the <u>Shrinrin-yoku</u> website.

## Music as a sleep-inducer

Music has been suggested as a soothing means of helping pregnant women to get to sleep and improve their quality of sleep each night. But is this something everyone can use, in terms of music, that can benefit all of us? Seems there may be an answer here.

Music, according to multiple research studies over the past several decades, has the ability to reduce nervous system activity, decrease anxiety, blood pressure, heart and respiratory rates and may have, in many cases, positive effects on sleep. The effects are primarily via muscle relaxation and distraction from disturbing thoughts you may have. In other words, music helps you to calm down in many ways and it is a beneficial asset for inducing sleep.

In fact, reports have shown that music has a statistically significant sleep-promoting effect and there is a significant decrease in depressive symptoms that may have been related to a lack of sleep. One note should be made here. While music is beneficial in bringing soothing sleep to you, listening to audiobooks was seen as having no effect and *was not recommended* as a sleep-inducing modality.

One study with students, who listened to calming classical music for 45 minutes at bedtime for three weeks, indicated that there was improvement in their ability to achieve restful sleep and, in fact, the improvement continued and increased during the third week of the study. The positive effect was seen to be via muscle relaxation and, again, freedom from distracting thoughts.

An interesting aspect that has been found in several studies is that the heart rate of individuals may slow down and synchronize with the musical beat being listened to. It is believed that this slowing may contribute to the relaxing effect of the music.

Another research finding was that students who listen to 45 minutes of music before bedtime, i.e., music of their own choosing, had a positive effect on multiple measures of sleep efficiency and it was seen as a means to prevent insomnia. Even when the music was of this self-selected type and not meditative classical music, it was effective in helping the students shorten sleep cycles and reach REM sleep more quickly.

The question of whether some types of music might be more effective than others was tackled in a study where they reported on 14 different musical genres comprising 545 artists and the results were the same; music was effective in bringing on sleep. Therefore, you can choose your sleep music as you wish.

One has to wonder, however, if very upbeat and fast tempo music would be a good choice and the researchers have not addressed this specific issue. Primarily, they indicate that music blocks external and internal stimuli that may disrupt sleep.

Music sleep studies have not been confined to young or student populations but have included a wide range of ages, musicality, sleep habits and stress levels. The conclusion, therefore, is that music is appropriate for all.

We can't deny that music does have the ability to calm us down and it has been proven to lower the stress hormone, cortisol, as well as induce a calming state. One neuroscience study reported that music can reduce anxiety levels as much as 65% which is quite impressive. When you are searching for something soothing to help you to sleep, it would appear that music is one thing to consider.

As in everything else, before you jump to the aggressive solutions, think of the simpler ones, like music for sleep. It's free, non-prescription and has even been found useful in *helping persons in chronic pain* to get a more restful night's sleep.

One musician who has produced eight-hours of music intended to calm and to assist you into getting to sleep, Max Richter has a selection on iTunes. Of course, it's not free, but might be worth the purchase if, after you sample it, you find it helpful. It's at: https://itunes.apple.com/us/album/sleep/id1020881374

*Remember, find the music that is **appropriate for you**. Several suggestions for music include:*

Rodrigo: Concierto de Aranjuez for Guitar and Orchestra - 2. Adagio
Miloš Karadaglić - RODRIGO: Concierto de Aranjuez - II. Adagio 10
    min. version
Aranjuez (Mon Amour)
"Watermark," by Enya (one I think is quite suitable)
"Canzonetta Sull'aria," by Mozart
"Someone Like You," by Adele
"Please Don't Go," by Barcelona
"Mellomaniac (Chill Out Mix)," by DJ Shah
"Electra," by Airstream
Johnny Mathis—Killing Me Softly with Her Song
Gregorian Monks Chants

A writer with an article on "Inc." has graciously placed a playlist of many of these musical selections on *Spotify*, which you can use free if you agree to ads. You might want to try it out at: https://open.spotify.com/playlist/71 mRGOhRHXZRSbQzouuFw7?si=wK9hoXHFQTm3RZELenxxOA.

There are also other classical musical selections that have been suggested as having calming effects on anyone who wants to drift off into dreamland, these include:

"Clair de Lune" by Claude Debussy
"Canzonetta Sul-aria" by Mozart
"Nocturne in E flat Major Op.9 No.2" by Chopin

If you'd like to try something truly different, and somewhat related to music because it depends on rhythm, there's a very good video on Youtube. In the video, musician Jim Donovan discusses how he finally got to sleep seven hours a night. For Jim it was either learn to slow down and sleep or shorten his life; he chose to live and he found his own method.

Previously, he had only been sleeping four hours a night, drank massive amounts of an energy drink and coffee and ended up in the hospital for three days. The hospital was where he got the bad news, sleep or die prematurely. So, he was more-than-urged to make critical changes in his life. The tapping and breathing exercise was only one of them.

What did he use? Something called *frequency patterning* which means our brains follow patterns. If we set the pace, our brain follows along and we can slow it down to a sleep-inducing state, which he successfully did. Certain music will all set the heart to follow the beat. A selection with a slow beat, therefore, should be more relaxing than a faster.

Of course, Donovan's method has many characteristics of <u>relaxation breathing</u> with an addition of tapping. It's worth a try, but as he indicates in his video, don't give up if one try doesn't do the trick. Keep at it for at least three nights because, as in so many things, practice is needed.

## Naps as a memory aid

Naps have received notice from researchers and not all of it points to naps being suggested for everyone. In fact, some researchers advise against napping because it may interfere with nighttime sleep. But others find that mid-day naps, something called *"power naps,"* can be very helpful in memory consolidation. Naps, in fact, may act as a daytime brain clearing mechanism.

We already know that sleep consolidates memory so it's best to read or work on something right before you nap. This pre-sleep activity puts information into short-term memory and then sleep comes along and moves it permanently into long-term memory. Just what you want.

If naps can be used during the daytime to prepare for later long-term memory storage at night, they would be encouraged. What should you do? When in doubt, test it out for yourself. We're not all made from the same mold.

## Plants as a relaxation aid

One additional thing which may not have occurred to you, but which is currently being shown interest by the scientific community, is the presence of plants in your sleep area. Plants, in general, are thought to clean the air and provide oxygen, but they have another potentially untapped use—a calming effect.

Unusual as it may sound, the CDC and the American Sleep Association have found a relationship between plants and sleep and, as a matter of fact, NASA conducted research studies where sleep and plants of a certain type, were investigated.

It appears just seeing the color green, unusual as that may seem, has a relaxing effect on us. Perhaps it is because it's often associated with outdoor green spaces where we are relaxed and this unconscious connection helps us to, once again, enter a state of relaxation. Some specific plants which have been found to be of interest to researchers and persons who believe that plants participate in some way in our sleep. They suggest the following:

lavender – seen to lower blood pressure and heart rate

jasmine – appears to help decrease anxiety and heighten mental performance

aloe vera – improves air quality because it absorbs certain microbes and other harmful particles which could disturb sleep

English ivy – helpful in reducing allergies as well as airborne mold by as much as 78% in 12 hours.

peace Lily – is also an air purifier and May put moisture into the air which can help with sinus and breathing difficulties related to dry, winter air.

Before bringing plants into your sleeping spaces, it is advisable that you consult with your primary care physician about this.

## Personal sleep logs/diaries

There are a number of things which encompass sleep hygiene and I've listed them already. But The American Academy of Sleep Medicine also has a very useful two-week sleep diary form that can be used to keep a record of your sleep activities.

Personal logs regarding what has happened during the week, when you went to sleep, and a few other items may direct you to more positive ways to get the sleep you need. A link where you may still find some of these downloadable diaries is at http://yoursleep.aasmnet.org/pdf/sleepdiary.pdf

The National Sleep Foundation provides an even more elaborate and fact-filled diary for you to download. The diary is quite inclusive and looks at all aspects of your activities prior to preparing for sleep each evening. Prepared like a visual diary, you may be more inclined to use this one because it is so complete. Go to their website (https://sleepfoundation.org) and download it.

You've gotten quite a few tips just a few pages ago (and you really should print them out), but more is better here, so here's more on sleep hygiene essentials and those who have a different take on it.

What are we hearing from other sleep researchers? They, for the most part, offer a few important tips that you may find beneficial. Remember, everyone is different and sleep habits may need adjustment to fit your biological needs, so consider each of the following and see how it might fit for you.

## Relaxation breathing

I have provided a video on Youtube.com where I explain and <u>demonstrate relaxation breathing.</u>

It's simple, you can learn it in minutes and practice it anywhere you happen to be; at work, at home, in the morning, at night or at a traffic light while your car is stopped. You can shorten it by just doing a few breaths and do a longer session later on. In fact, if you're in an elevator and you have an important meeting to which you're going, do some relaxation breathing. And, of course, try it before you go to bed. The sense of calm you will feel has been compared to taking a pill, but it's much more *under your control*.

## Rocking

Wouldn't it be wonderful if we could find something that was both soothing and helped us quickly get to sleep? Thankfully, there is something and we've been using it all along, but not as adults. We limited it to children or to persons in distress. What is it? Rocking.

Children, as we all know, enjoy rocking as a soothing activity which is often used to help them to get to sleep or to calm down after one of their minor accidents. The action of rocking, in fact, seems to come naturally to us as we hold others who are feeling emotional pain. We attempt to help them heal and handle this by gently rocking them as we hold them in our arms.

The action of rocking would seem to have some intimate connection to our biology and to personal soothing. Not only does this appear to be apparent to the casual observer, but it has been observed in research studies that have shown rocking is an effective way to help you get to sleep and improve memory.

Studies have shown that rocking does help us get to sleep, but also to maintain sleep and has an effect on enhancing memory formation during sleep. Deep within our brains the rocking sets off some as-yet unknown pathway to reinforce things we wish to memorize. You've probably noticed that rocking cribs and rocking chairs are coming back into use as people sense the value in rocking.

Technical hookups have gauged rocking's significant effect and how it brings about changes in brainwave activity related to this rocking behavior. Interestingly enough, rocking overnight is related not just to memory improvement but it is believed that this is involved in changing brain-wave activity which is beneficial for our memory consolidation. But how does an adult or even a child maintain all-night rocking?

Beds, of course, could be constructed, as they were in experiments on rocking and sleep, to produce a gentle rocking movement. The advent, some three or four decades ago, of waterbeds may have unknowingly tapped into the benefits of rocking as any movement in the bed would provide a gentle swaying movement beneath us.

Delving further into how or what rocking might do, researchers found that not only did rocking shorten the time to go to sleep, it also strengthens deep sleep which is helpful in maintaining rest. Perrault at al. (2019), in their study of rocking and sleep, indicated that, "*Taken together, the present findings demonstrate that applying a rhythmic sensory stimulation... using a rocking bed during a whole night of sleep, promotes deep sleep and memory consolidation in healthy sleepers.*" It was the opinion of these researchers that, "*These results may be relevant to the development of non-pharmacological therapies for patients with insomnia or mood disorders, or even for aging populations who frequently suffer from decreased sleep and/or from memory impairments."*

Rocking, undoubtedly, is now a proven, scientific way to achieve better sleep and enhanced learning for students or anyone wishing to have a more robust ability to remember something.

### The FOMO phenomenon

Digital media, in particular smartphones, have invaded our lives and, in so doing, created an atmosphere of anxiety and sleep disruption. How did this happen and what is FOMO, anyway? The acronym FOMO stands for "Fear of Missing Out" and it accounts for quite a bit of lost sleep.

If I don't check my phone regularly, these individuals with FOMO believe, I may miss something important, I won't be included, people will think I don't care, etc. The list goes on as long as the anxiety that drives it. The Baby Boomers appear to be at greatest risk for developing this problem.

The perceived belief that connectedness is vital at all hours leads to higher levels of anxiety, which, in turn, leads to a loss of valuable sleep time. One researcher asked if our wireless technology might be creating a new class of disorders he named "*iDisorders.*" Good question and researchers are fervently seeking answers. Digital devices were one of the factors which Rosen and other have suggested could be contributing to disorders where pre-existing psychiatric conditions, not yet diagnosed, were present.

### Things to consider at bedtime

Okay, what about the old standby, milk? Ever hear of someone suggesting a nice glass of warm milk to help you get to sleep? Do you know how much milk you'd have to consume in order to really get its sleep-inducing properties to work for you? The ingredient in milk that induces sleep is *tryptophan* and it's also found in turkey.

I've heard you've had to drink somewhere around *8 glasses* to get the sleep benefit from warm milk. I don't think you want to down a quart or more of milk right before you go to bed.

*Daytime light* is not to be avoided but included as another thing to put into your sleep routine. So, try to go for a walk outside if it's sunny. It can help in ways we never imagined. Natural light helps the sleep-wake cycle stay tuned up and it also *helps with Vitamin D* which may help fight depression.

Once you are in bed, provide yourself with a *serene scene* and imagine yourself there. Concentrate on it, the scents, the location and allow yourself to fall completely into it. It's a bit of self-hypnosis and that's fine. Right now, you have only one task and that's to help yourself relax and sleep. Tomorrow will come soon enough.

A few more tips on sleep hygiene center around keeping your bed the place you sleep as has been stressed in this book. Bed is not the place you do work, eat meals, work on the computer or watch TV. And, let's not forget that you want *shades on the windows* to provide as much darkness as possible. Yes, you can buy special shades for your bedroom that have the ability to block unwanted light.

The temperature of your bedroom is important, too, and it's best to have it cool in addition to the room being quiet.

If, for whatever reason, you don't begin to practice good sleep hygiene habits, you may well experience sleep deprivation. How will that play out? Well, in truly unpleasant, unhealthy and upsetting ways.

You'll be sleepy during the day, grouchy and finding yourself lacking in motivation and creativity. Doesn't matter what you do during your day because everything will be affected whether you work or remain in the home.

No getting away from it and it's like an invisible illness you carry around with you and with little help from anyone. You are the one who has the power here, so use it and benefit by that use.

If you ever feel yourself questioning whether or not you should sacrifice sleep on a regular basis, also question yourself about the illnesses you may develop. What is worth more than your health? Doesn't it make sense to protect it?

## What to avoid at bedtime

As you've already read, stimulants such as *caffeine, nicotine or alcohol*, as we know, are definitely to be avoided when you're getting ready for bed. Yet, I knew a very famous actor who told me that he couldn't get to sleep at night without a bottle or two of wine. He had quite a fine cellar in his West Side Manhattan triplex and he tapped it nightly to bring on sleep. Without the wine, he said, he just couldn't get to sleep. It was in his later years and I wondered whether he had a drinking problem.

*Alcohol*, as I've indicated, may initially help with the feeling of sleepiness but later in the night it can lead to arousal. The next day you can wake up not only poorly rested, but with a bit of depression as well.

*Exercise* before going to bed is not a good idea, either. Experts tell us that, while exercise during the morning or earlier in the day does help with sleep, it can be too stimulating just before bedtime. The only form of exercise which may be useful is yoga and not just before bedtime.

## Tips for employers:

Employers can consider adjusting work schedules to allow their workers time to get enough sleep (or take naps?).

Employers can also educate their shiftworkers about how to improve their sleep. Employers also should realize that drowsy or sleep-deprived employees are not as creative or possibly even as invested in their projects and cost corporations money in lost hours of work for sickness, injuries, higher healthcare costs, disability insurance for these accidents on the job and efficiency. If a company wants creative employees who'll meet their work deadlines, they need proper sleep. Sleep and making any work adjustments to ensure adequate sleep is in everyone's best interest.

# AFTERWORD

Sleep is a topic that is both intriguing and vexing because so much is unknown and there's still a lot of people out there who think they can easily get by on less sleep even in the face of research that has shown they can't. The consequences for denying the obvious will be known to them but they may never suspect it was all because they failed to adhere to a sensible sleep schedule.

I don't know if you can convince them otherwise, even if you loan them this book. They think they have to keep busy and sleep is a waste of time. Do you think it's a waste of time or have your eyes been opened to what sleep really does and how important it is to your health? What about the key to creativity that sleep provides when that right hemisphere gets into gear? Don't you want access to that? Of course, you do.

I hope you've found this book useful and that you will share it with others. Sleep tight tonight and don't forget those wonderful, refreshing and creativity-enhancing naps.

Written on the beaches of Sanibel Island (in my dreams).

# ABOUT THE AUTHOR

Dr. Patricia A. Farrell is a well-known licensed psychologist, WebMD consultant, a consultant to pharmaceutical firms, published author of multiple self-help books and videos, former medical consultant for Social Security Disability Determinations, psychiatric researcher at Mt. Sinai Medical Center (NYC) and an educator who has taught on the college as well as graduate and post-graduate levels. Dr. Farrell has appeared on such national TV shows as The Today Show, The View, Court TV, MSNBC, AC360, CNN, HLN, VH1, MTV, ABC World News, Voice of America and on international, regional and national syndicated radio as well as in print media in national newspapers and magazines.

Dr. Farrell is a biographee in Who's Who in the World, Who's Who in America and Who's Who of American Women. A member of The American Psychological Association as well as the SAG-AFTRA union, she is a former board member of the New Jersey Board of Psychological Examiners as well as a former board of directors' member of Bergen Pines Hospital in New Jersey and was a psychiatry preceptor at The University of Medicine & Dentistry of New Jersey.

# REFERENCES

Adams, J. U. (2019, February 09). What you need to know about sleep medications, their side effects and other issues. Retrieved from https://wapo.st/2I6Hnco

Acsády, L., & Harris, K. D. (2017). Synaptic scaling in sleep. Science, 355(6324), 457-457.

Adult Stem Cells Activated In Mammalian Brain. (2008, July 26). Retrieved from https://www.sciencedaily.com/releases/2008/07/080724150437.htm

Alcohol Use in Older People. (2012). National Institute on Aging.

Allen, M. (n.d.). You Snooze, You Lose: Insurers Make the Old Adage Literally True. Retrieved from https://www.propublica.org/article/you-snooze-you-lose-insurers-make-the-old-adage-literally-true

Ambien: Does This Popular Sleep Medication Turn People into Zombies? (n.d.). Retrieved from https://www.ajpb.com/news/ambien-does-this-popular-sleep-medication-turn-people-into-zombies

American Psychological Association (2016). Why sleep is important and what happens if you don't get enough. http://www.apa.org/topics/sleep/why.aspx

Amy, H, Keage, D., Banks, S., Yang, K. et al. (2012). What sleep characteristics predict cognitive decline in the elderly? Sleep Medicine, 13(7), 886-892.

André, C. (2019, January 15). Proper Breathing Brings Better Health. Retrieved from https://www.scientificamerican.com/article/proper-breathing-brings-better-health/

Ann, M. A., & Banerjee, M. (2016). Melatonin Disruption in Autism and Its Regulation by Natural Supplements. Serotonin and Melatonin, 499-512.

Antony, J. W., Gobel, E. W., O'Hare, J. K., Reber, P. J., & Paller, K. A. (2012). Cued memory reactivation during sleep influences skill learning. Nature Neuroscience,15(8), 1114-1116.

Anwar, Y., & Anwar, Y. (2019, January 28). Sleep loss heightens pain sensitivity, dulls brain's painkilling response. Retrieved from https://news.berkeley.edu/2019/01/28/sleep-pain-connection/

Askitopoulou, H. (2015). Sleep and Dreams: From Myth to Medicine in Ancient Greece. Anesthesia History, 1(3), 70-75.

Askitopoulou, H. (2002). Surgical cures under sleep induction in the Asclepieion of Epidauros. International Congress Series, v.1242, December 11-17.

Auerbach, S., & Yaffe, K. (2016). The link between sleep-disordered breathing and cognition in the elderly. Neurology,88(5), 424-425.

Axelsson, J., Sundelin, T., Ingre, M., Someren, E. J., Olsson, A., & Lekander, M. (2010, December 15). Beauty sleep: Experimental study on the perceived health and attractiveness of sleep deprived people. British Medical Journal, 341:c6614. Retrieved from https://www.bmj.com/content/341/bmj.c6614

Baptiste, N. (1995). Adults need to play, too. Early Childhood Education Journal, 23(1), 33-35.

Barger, L. K., Flynn-Evans, E. E., Kubey, A., Walsh, L., Ronda, J. M. et al. (2014). Prevalence of sleep deficiency and use of hypnotic drugs in astronauts before, during, and after spaceflight: An observational study. *The Lancet Neurology,13*(9), 904-912.

Barros, V. V., Martins, L. F., Saitz, R., Bastos, R. R., & Ronzani, T. M. (2012). Mental health conditions, individual and job characteristics and sleep disturbances among firefighters. Journal of Health Psychology, 18(3), 350-358.

Behrman, S., Ebmeier, K. (2014). Can exercise prevent cognitive decline? Practitioner, 258(1767), 17-21.

Berkman, L. F., Buxton, O., Ertel, K., & Okechukwu, C. (2010). Managers' practices related to work–family balance predict employee cardiovascular risk and sleep duration in extended care settings. Journal of Occupational Health Psychology, 15(3), 316-329.

Bernert, R. A. (2014, October 01). Poor Sleep Quality as a Risk Factor for Suicide. Retrieved from https://jamanetwork.com/journals/jamapsychiatry/fullarticle/1895670

Black, D. S., O'Reilly, G. A., Olmstead, R., Breen, E. C., & Irwin, M. R. (2015). Mindfulness Meditation and Improvement in Sleep Quality and Daytime Impairment Among Older Adults with Sleep Disturbances. JAMA Internal Medicine JAMA Intern Med, 175(4), 494.

Blue light has a dark side. (2012, May). Harvard Health Letter. Retrieved February 14from http://www.health.harvard.edu/staying-healthy/blue-light-has-a-dark-side.

Bowen, J. (2019, April 11). Sleep Apnea and Dementia: What's the Connection ... Retrieved from https://www.neurologytimes.com/aan/sleep-apnea-and-dementia-whats-connection

Breus, M. (2018, May 01). How Sleep Deprivation Hurts Your Emotional Health. Retrieved from https://thesleepdoctor.com/2018/05/01/how-sleep-deprivation-hurts-your-emotional-health/

Breus, M. (2010, April). Sleep Violence: Rare, but Real « Sleep Well. Retrieved February 22, 2017, from http://blogs.webmd.com/sleep-disorders/2010/04/sleep-violence-rare-but-real.html

Brooks, M. FDA Adds Boxed Warning to Insomnia Drugs. Medscape, April 30, 2019.

Brunk, D. (2015, November). Shorter sleep linked to faster kidney function decline. Retrieved February 23, 2016, from http://www.internalmedicinenews.com/specialty-focus/nephrology/single-article-page/shorter-sleep-linked-to-faster-kidney-function-decline/b29d97d05778aa89f919a30fdbbc2b9d.html

Buchanan, D. T., Landis, C. A., Hohensee, C., Guthrie, K. A., Otte, J. L., Paudel, M., Ensrud, K. E. (2017). Effects of Yoga and Aerobic Exercise on Actigraphic Sleep Parameters in Menopausal Women with Hot Flashes. Journal of Clinical Sleep Medicine,13(01), 11-18.

Butler, C. (2010, June 29). Circadian rhythms are powerful, but people can change their sleep-wake cycles. Washingtonpost.com.

Buxton, O. M., Cain, S. W., O'Connor, S. P., Porter, J. H., Duffy, J. F., Wang, W., Shea, S. A. (2012). Adverse Metabolic Consequences in Humans of Prolonged Sleep Restriction Combined with Circadian Disruption. Science Translational Medicine, 4(129).

Buxton, O. M., & Shea, S. A. (2018 Dec; 4(6)). Sleep & work, work & sleep. Sleep Health,497-498.

Capretto, L. (2015, August 04). Think Drinking Alcohol Before Bed Can Help You Sleep? Not Even Close. Retrieved from https://www. huffpost.com/entry/drinking-alcohol-sleep-impact_n_55bba1b4e4b0d 4f33a02923e

Carpenter, S. (2011). Awakening to sleep. Stress & Health, 27(4), 314-324. Retrieved February 15, 2016.

Carskadon, M. Brown, E & Dement, W. (1982). Sleep fragmentation in the elderly: Relationship to daytime sleep tendency. Neurobiology of Aging, 3, 321-327.

Castillo, S. (2016). Sleep-Deprived People Are More Likely to Crave Junk Food. Medical Daily. Retrieved March 01, 2016, from http://www. medicaldaily.com/sleep- deprivation-weight-gain-munchies-375684

Centers for Disease Control and Prevention (2016, January 4). Attention-Deficit / Hyperactivity Disorder (ADHD) New Data: Medication and Behavior Treatment. Retrieved February 27, 2016, from http://www. cdc.gov/ncbddd/adhd/data.html

Centers for Disease Control (2015). NIOSH Training for Nurses on Shift Work and Long Work Hours. CDC Course Numbers: WB2408 and WB2409. Retrieved from http://www.cdc.gov/niosh/docs/2015-115/

Centers for Disease Control (2013). Prescription Sleep Aid Use Among Adults: United States, 2005–2010. NCHS Data Brief, 127, August. http://www.cdc.gov/nchs/data/databriefs/db127.htm#x2013;2010

Centers for Disease Control (2015). Therapeutic Drug Use. FastStats. http://www.cdc.gov/nchs/fastats/drug-use-therapeutic.htm

Cheever, N. A., Rosen, L. D., Carrier, L. M., & Chavez, A. (2014). Out of sight is not out of mind: The impact of restricting wireless mobile device use on anxiety levels among low, moderate and high users. Computers in Human Behavior,37, 290-297.

Chelala, Cesar (2013). What's the point in working yourself to death? The Japan Times, January 7. Retrieved from http://www.japantimes.co.jp/ opinion/2013/01/07/commentary/world- commentary/whats-the-point-in-working-yourself-to-death/.

Chen, H., Hsu, N., & Chou, P. (2017). The Association between Sleep Duration and Hand Grip Strength in Community-Dwelling Older Adults: The Yilan Study, Taiwan. Sleep.

Cimons, M. (1991). Halcion Sleeping Pill Banned by Britain; Risks Seen. LA Times. Retrieved from https://www.latimes.com/archives/la-xpm-1991-10-03-mn-4409-story.html

Cohen, D. A., Wang, W., Wyatt, J. K., Kronauer, R. E., Dijk, D., Czeisler, C. A., & Klerman, E. B. (2010). Uncovering Residual Effects of Chronic Sleep Loss on Human Performance. Science Translational Medicine, 2(14).

Cohen, S. (2014). The lasting legacy of a case that was lost. Retrieved February 17, 2016, from http://www.pennstatelawreview.org/wp-content/uploads/2014/09/Cohen_The-Lasting-Legacy-of-a-Case-that-was- Lost.pdf

Colvin, G. (2015) Do Successful CEOs Sleep Less Than Everyone Else? Fortune, November 18. Retrieved from http://fortune.com/2015/11/18/sleep-habits-donald- trump/.

Coren, S. (1998). Sleep deprivation, psychosis and mental efficiency. Psychiatric Times, 15(3). Retrieved February 27, 2016 from http://www.psychiatrictimes.com/articles/sleep-deprivation-psychosis-and-mental- efficiency

Crum, Alia J., and Ellen J. Langer. 2007. Mind-set matters: Exercise and the placebo effect. Psychological Science 18, no. 2: 165-171.

Cruz, J. (2010). Zolpidem and Uncontrollable Nocturnal Eating Binges. Clinical Correlations. Langone NYU Journal of Medicine, February 24. Retrieved from http://www.clinicalcorrelations.org/?p=2345

Centers for Disease Control and Prevention (2006). Fatalities among volunteer and career firefighters--United States, 1994-2004. Retrieved from https://www.cdc.gov/mmwr/preview/mmwrhtml/mm5516a3.htm

Corbley, A. (2018, September 04). Put These 5 Plants in Your Bedroom Window for a Better Night's Sleep. Retrieved from https://www.goodnewsnetwork.org/put-these-5-plants-in-your-bedroom-window-for-a-better-nights-sleep/

Cupp, M. (1999). Herbal Remedies: Adverse Effects and Drug Interactions. American Family Physician. March 1, 59(5),1239-1244. Retrieved from http://www.aafp.org/afp/1999/0301/p1239.html

Curtin, M. (2017, May 30). Neuroscience Says Listening to This Song Reduces Anxiety by Up to 65 Percent. Retrieved from https://www.inc.com/melanie-curtin/neuroscience-says-listening-to-this-one-song-reduces-anxiety-by-up-to-65-percent.html

Darwin, C. (2009). Origin of species: 150th anniversary edition. Alachua, FL: Bridge-Logos.

Davenport, L. (2019, April 15). Melatonin Benefits Kids With Autism, Ups Parents' Quality of Life. Retrieved from https://www.medscape.com/viewarticle/911804

Davidson, J., Mendis, J., Stuck, A. R., DeMichele, G., & Zisook, S. (2018, August 17). Nurse Suicide: Breaking the Silence. Retrieved from https://nam.edu/nurse-suicide-breaking-the-silence/

Dawson, J. (2016). Putting the brakes on drowsy driving, The American Nurse, February 16. Retrieved from http://www.theamericannurse.org/index.php/2012/04/02/putting-the-brakes-on- drowsy-driving/

Dawson, V. (2016). Supporting young people with sleep issues to meet their full potential. Education and Health, 34(4).

Depner, C. M., Melanson, E. L., Eckel, R. H., Snell-Bergeon, J. K., & Perreault, L. (2019). Ad libitum Weekend Recovery Sleep Fails to Prevent Metabolic Dysregulation during a Repeating Pattern of Insufficient Sleep and Weekend Recovery Sleep. Current Biology.

Derickson, A. (2014). Dangerously sleepy: Overworked Americans and the cult of manly wakefulness. Philadelphia: University of Pennsylvania Press.

Delayed Sleep Phase Syndrome (DSPS) in Children and Adolescents. (n.d.). Retrieved from https://my.clevelandclinic.org/health/diseases/14295-delayed-sleep-phase-syndrome-dsps-in-children-and-adolescents

Devlin, H. (2015, June 5). Newly discovered vessels beneath skull could link brain and the immune system. The Guardian.com. Retrieved February 27, 2016 from http://www.theguardian.com/science/2015/jun/05/newly-discovered-vessels- beneath-skull-could-link-brain-and-immune-system

Dillon, J., & Chervin, R. (2012, June 13). ADHD and Sleep Disorders in Children. Psychiatric Times. Retrieved February 27, 2016, from http://www.psychiatrictimes.com/adhd/adhd-and-sleep-disorders-children

Dion, K., Berscheid, E., & Walster, E. (1972). What is beautiful is good. Journal of personality and social psychology, 24, 285-290

Doyle, K. (2016, August 03). Memory may someday benefit from electric therapy. Retrieved from https://www.reuters.com/article/us-health-brain-stimulation-sleep-idUSKCN10E219

Doyle, L. (1987). Medical Experts Seek Clues to 'Nightmare Deaths' That Strike Male Asian Refugees. UPI, January 11.

Drake, C. (2014). Shift Work and Sleep. National Sleep Foundation. Retrieved March 2, 2016, from https://sleepfoundation.org/sleep-topics/shift-work-and-sleep

Draganich, C., & Erdal, K. (2014). Placebo sleep affects cognitive functioning. Journal of Experimental Psychology: Learning, Memory, and Cognition,40(3), 857-864.

Dreyfuss, E. (2019, April 19). You're Not Getting Enough Sleep-and It's Killing You. Retrieved from https://www.wired.com/story/youre-not-getting-enough-sleep-and-its-killing-you/

Ducharme, J. (2018, May 30). Time Magazine. Roseanne Barr used the 'Ambien Defense.' So have accused murderers and drunk drivers. Retrieved from http://bitly.com/2WRXZb5

Ducharme, J. (2014, June 17). How white noise helps us sleep. Boston Magazine. Retrieved from http://www.bostonmagazine.com/health/blog/2014/06/17/white- noise/

Duffy, J. , Wilson, H, Wang, W., & Czeisler, C. (2009). Healthy older adults better tolerate Sleep deprivation than younger adults. Journal of American Geriatric Society, July 57(7), 1245-1251.

Duke-NUS Medical School. (2017, January 9). Association between insufficient sleep, gestational diabetes mellitus discovered. ScienceDaily. Retrieved from www.sciencedaily.com/releases/2017/01/170109092634.htm

Durmer, J. & Dinges, D. (2005). Neurocognitive consequences of sleep deprivation. In K. Roos (Ed.) Sleep in Neurological Practice. Seminars in Neurology, 25(1), 117- 129.

Early pregnancy shifts body clock by a few hours. (2019, May 03). Retrieved from https://www.futurity.org/first-trimester-body-clock-pregnancy-2052162-2/?utm_source=Futurity Today&utm_campaign= 24df466934-

Eating at 'wrong time' affects body weight, circadian rhythms. (2017, July 18). Retrieved from https://www.sciencedaily.com/ releases/2017/07/170718091542.htm

Electronics in the Bedroom: Why it's Necessary to Turn off Before You Tuck in. Retrieved from https://sleepfoundation.org/ask-the- expert/ electronics-the-bedroom

Erickson, M. H., Rosen, S., Erickson, M. H., & Erickson, M. H. (1991). My voice will go with you: the teaching tales of Milton H. Erickson. New York: W.W. Norton.

Erlacher, C., Erlacher, D., & Schredl, M. (2015). The effects of exercise on self-rated sleep among adults with chronic sleep complaints. Journal of Sport and Health Science, 4(3), 289-298.

Erland, L. A., & Saxena, P. K. (2017). Melatonin Natural Health Products and Supplements: Presence of Serotonin and Significant Variability of Melatonin Content. Journal of Clinical Sleep Medicine,13(02), 275-281.

Euston, D. R., & Steenland, H. W. (2014). Memories--getting wired during sleep. Science, 344(6188), 1087-1088.

Eveleth, R. (2014, January 22). You Can Get Placebo Sleep. http:// www.smithsonianmag.com/smart-news/you-can-get-placebo-sleep-180949410/

Ferracioli-Oda, E., Qawasmi, A., & Bloch, M. H. (2013). Meta-Analysis: Melatonin for the Treatment of Primary Sleep Disorders. PLoS ONE,8(5).

Forest Bathing - What It Is and How it Helps Stress. (2018, August 09). Retrieved from https://www.amerisleep.com/blog/forest-bathing-stress/

Freud, S., & Brill, A. A. (1997). The interpretation of dreams. Hertfordshire, UK: Wordsworth Classics of World Literature.

Fryer, B. (2006). Sleep deficit: The performance killer. A conversation with Professor Charles A. Czeisler. Harvard Business Review, October 84(10), 53-9, 148. Retrieved from https://hbr.org/2006/10/sleep-deficit-the-performance-killer

Gander, P., & Signal, L. (2008). Who Is Too Old for Shift Work? Developing Better Criteria. Chronobiology International, 25(2-3), 199-213.

Garke, M. & Svensson, I. (n.d.) Sleep in and get the job: An experimental study on the relationship between sleep restriction and perceived employability. Retrieved from http://bitly.com/2QVVSDD.

Global Obesity. (2012). American Journal of Human Biology, 24(3), 361-371.

Greusel, John (1913). Thomas Edison: The man, the work and his mind. (Arts & Crafts). https://books.google.com/books?id=ak4yAQAAMAAJ&printsec=frontcover#v=one page&q&f=false

Grinde, B., & Patil, G. (2009). Biophilia: Does Visual Contact with Nature Impact on Health and Well-Being? International Journal of Environmental Research and Public Health,6(9), 2332-2343.

Gulia KK and Kumar VM. Sleep Deprivation during pregnancy: The Cost of Ignorance!. SM J Sleep Disorders. 2016; 2(1): 1004.

Hamilton, J. (2018, August 27). What Makes A Human Brain Unique? A Newly Discovered Neuron May Be A Clue. Retrieved from https://www.npr.org/sections/health-shots/2018/08/27/642255886/a-new-discovery-may-explain-what-makes-the-human-brain-unique

Hanlon, E. C., Tasali, E., Leproult, R., Stuhr, K. L., Doncheck, E., Wit, H. D., Cauter, E. V. (2016). Sleep Restriction Enhances the Daily Rhythm of Circulating Levels of Endocannabinoid 2-Arachidonoylglycerol. Sleep, 39(03), 653-664.

Harmat, L., Takács, J., & Bódizs, R. (2008, May). Music improves sleep quality in students. Retrieved from https://www.ncbi.nlm.nih.gov/pubmed/18426457/

Hearne, K. M. (1982). Effects Of Performing Certain Set Tasks In The Lucid-Dream State. Perceptual and Motor Skills, 54(1), 259-262.

Helping Your Child With Autism Get a Good Night's Sleep. (2018, May 20). Retrieved from https://www.webmd.com/brain/autism/helping-your-child-with-autism-get-a-good-nights-sleep

Holloway, K. (2016, February 23). Having to Work Before 10 AM Is 'Torture,' Scientist Says. Retrieved from http://www.alternet.org/ personal- health/having-work-10-am-torture-scientist-says.

Holst, H. M., & Kerkhof, G. A. (2014). Shift work tolerance and the importance of sleep quality: A study of police officers. Biological Rhythm Research, 46(2), 257-264.

Horne JA and Östberg O. (1976) A self-assessment questionnaire to determine morningness-eveningness in human circadian rhythms. International Journal of Chronobiology. 4:97-100.

How do we hear while we sleep? Science Daily (April 30, 1998). Retrieved from https://www.sciencedaily.com/releases/1998/04/980430044534. htm

Howell, E. (2014, August 14). Astronauts Are Sleep-Deprived in Space. Retrieved from https://www.space.com/26829-astronauts-space-station-sleep-deprivation.html

Hsiao, Y., Chen, Y., Tseng, C., Wu, L., Lin, W., et al. (2015). Sleep Disorders and Increased Risk of Autoimmune Diseases in Individuals without Sleep Apnea. Sleep, 2015; 38(4), 581–586.

Huang, G. & Stapczynski, S. (October 19, 2016) Suicide of overworked woman, 24, prompts ad giant Dentsu to trim overtime hours. The Japan Times. http://www.japantimes.co.jp/news/2016/10/19/business/ suicide-overworked-woman-24-prompts-ad-giant-dentsu-trim-overtime-hours/#.WLtULBLytDU

Hui, F. K. (2015). Clearing Your Mind: A Glymphatic System? World Neurosurgery,83(5), 715-717.

Hui, S. A., & Grandner, M. A. (2015). Associations between poor sleep quality and stages of change of multiple health behaviors among participants of employee wellness program. Preventive Medicine Reports, 2, 292-299.

Ingravallo, F., Poli, F., Gilmore, E. V., Pizza, F., Vignatelli, L., Schenck, C. H., & Plazzi, G. (2014). Sleep-Related Violence and Sexual Behavior in Sleep: A Systematic Review of Medical-Legal Case Reports. Journal of Clinical Sleep Medicine.

Irwin, M. R., Olmstead, R., & Carroll, J. E. (2016). Sleep Disturbance,

Sleep Duration, and Inflammation: A Systematic Review and Meta-Analysis of Cohort Studies and Experimental Sleep Deprivation. Biological Psychiatry,80(1), 40-52.

Irwin, M., Wang, M., Ribeiro, D., Cho, H., Olmstead, R., et al. (2008). Sleep loss activates cellular inflammatory signaling. Biological Psychiatry, 64(6), September 538-540.

Ives, J. (2019, April 08). Sleep disruption leads to negativity bias, study shows. Retrieved from https://www.news-medical.net/news/20190408/Sleep-disruption-leads-to-negativity-bias-study-shows.aspx

Jaffe, E. (2015, May 19). Morning people vs. night owls: 9 insights backed by science. Retrieved from https://www.fastcodesign.com/3046391/evidence/morning-people-vs-night-people-9-insights-backed-by-science

James, W. (2017). Hypnotics and the Risks of Dementia. *Journal of Clinical Sleep Medicine,13*(06), 837-837.

Jensen, T., Kold, T., Andersson, A., Anna-Maria, & Erik, N. (2013, April 07). Association of Sleep Disturbances With Reduced Semen Quality: A Cross-sectional Study Among 953 Healthy Young Danish Men. Retrieved from https://academic.oup.com/aje/article/177/10/1027/101677

Jonas, J. (2015, December 29). How a Good Night's Sleep - and a Bad Night's Sleep - Can Enhance Your Creativity. Retrieved from http://www.openculture.com/2015/12/sleep-and-creativity.html

John, M. W. (1991). A new method for measuring daytime sleepiness: The Epworth Sleepiness Scale. American Sleep Disorders Association and Sleep Research Society, 14(6), 540-545.

Juul, J. (2010). A casual revolution: Reinventing video games and their players. Cambridge, MA: MIT Press.

Karan, A. (2017, March 01). Do doctors' other motivations, like the need for sleep, affect patient care. https://yhoo.it/2I6FqN6

Kay-Stacey, M., & Attarian, H. P. (2017). Managing Sleep Disorders during Pregnancy. *Gender and the Genome*, 34–45.

Khazan, O. (2014). Thomas Edison and the Cult of Sleep Deprivation. The Atlantic. May 14. http://www.theatlantic.com/health/archive/2014/05/thomas-edison-and-the-cult-of- sleep-deprivation/370824/

Kleeman, J. (2017, March 04). 'I'll go to school on two and a half hours' sleep': Why British children aren't sleeping. Retrieved from https://www.theguardian.com/lifeandstyle/2017/mar/04/go-school-two-half-hours-sleep-british-children-arent-sleeping.

Klemm, W. (n.d.). How Sleep Helps Memory. Retrieved from https://www.psychologytoday.com/intl/blog/memory-medic/201103/how-sleep-helps-memory

Kotsovolis, G., & Komninos, G. (2009). Awareness during anesthesia: how sure can we be that the patient is sleeping indeed? *Hippokratia, 13*(2), 83–89.

Lantz, F., & Zimmerman, E. Rules, Play and Culture. Retrieved March 01, 2016, from http://www.ericzimmerman.com/texts/RulesPlayCulture.html

Lamberg, L. (n.d.). Short Sleep Duration Increases Adolescent Suicide Risk. https://psychnews.psychiatryonline.org/doi/10.1176/appi.pn.2018.11b24

Lee, H., Xie, L., Yu, M., Kang, H., Feng, T., Deane, R., Benveniste, H. (2015). The Effect of Body Posture on Brain Glymphatic Transport. Journal of Neuroscience, 35(31), 11034-11044.

Lee, Y., Park, J., Kim, S., Cho, S., & Kim, S. (2017, November 08). Study links insufficient sleep to poor academic performance among teens. Retrieved from https://aasm.org/study-links-insufficient-sleep-to-poor-academic-performance-among-teens/

Levinson, D. J. (1986). The Seasons of a Man's Life. New York: Ballantine Books.

Lewis, T. (2016, February 2). This one factor may explain why you're a morning person or a night owl. Business Insider. Retrieved from http://www.businessinsider.com/being-a-morning-person-or-a-night-owl-is-in-your- genes-2016-2

Linden, D. (2011, October 25). Video Games Can Activate the Brain's Pleasure Circuits. Retrieved from https://www.psychologytoday.com/blog/the-compass-pleasure/201110/video-games-can-activate-the-brains-pleasure-circuits- 0

Liu, R., Qian, Z., Trevathan, E., Chang, J., Zelicoff, A., Hao, Y., Dong, G. (2015). Poor sleep quality associated with high risk of hypertension and elevated blood pressure in China: Results from a large population-based study. Hypertension Research, 39(1), 54-59.

Lmunoz, L. (2019, March 26). Going Deep on Sleep with Matthew Walker. Retrieved from https://www.cogneurosociety.org/going-deep-sleep-matthew-walker/

Macedo, D. M., & Diez-Garcia, R. W. (2014). Sweet craving and ghrelin and leptin levels in women during stress. Appetite, 80, 264-270.

MacMillan, A. (2017, April 17). Teens May Do Better When School Starts Later. Retrieved from http://time.com/4741147/school-start-time/

Mann, D. (n.d.). Lack of Sleep and the Immune System. Retrieved from https://www.webmd.com/sleep-disorders/features/immune-system-lack-of-sleep

Mars, K. (2018, January 31). NASA Twins Study Confirms Changes to Mark Kelly's Genes. Retrieved from https://www.nasa.gov/feature/nasa-twins-study-confirms-preliminary-findings

Martin-Fairey, C. A., Zhao, P., Wan, L., Roenneberg, T., Fay, J., Ma, X., … Herzog, E. D. (2019). Pregnancy Induces an Earlier Chronotype in Both Mice and Women. Journal of Biological Rhythms. https://doi.org/10.1177/0748730419844650

McAlpine, C. S., Kiss, M. G., Rattik, S., He, S., Vassalli, A., Anzai, A., . . . Swirski, F. K. (2019, February 13). Sleep modulates haematopoiesis and protects against atherosclerosis. Retrieved from https://www.nature.com/articles/s41586-019-0948-2

McGuire, B. E., Basten, C. J., Ryan, C. J., & Gallagher, J. (2000). Intensive Care Unit Syndrome. Archives of Internal Medicine, 160(7), 906.

McMillan, F. (2019, February 13). How Sleep Fights Infection: Snoozing Makes Killer Immune Cells More Sticky. Retrieved from https://www.forbes.com/sites/fionamcmillan/2019/02/12/how-sleep-fights-infection-snoozing-makes-killer-immune-cells-more-sticky/

Merz, Beverly. "This Is Your Brain on Alcohol." Harvard Health Blog, 13 July 2017, www.health.harvard.edu/blog/this-is-your-brain-on-alcohol-2017071412000.

Morbidity and Mortality Weekly Report (2012), November 9, 61(44), 895-898. Energy Drink Consumption and Its Association with Sleep Problems Among U.S. Service Members on a Combat Deployment

— Afghanistan, 2010. Retrieved from http://www.cdc.gov/mmwr/preview/mmwrhtml/mm6144a3.htm

Murdock, K. K., Horissian, M., & Crichlow-Ball, C. (2016). Emerging Adults' Text Message Use and Sleep Characteristics: A Multimethod, Naturalistic Study. Behavioral Sleep Medicine, 1-14.

Music Psychology. (n.d.). Retrieved from http://musicpsychology.co.uk/music-and-sleep/

Naps Clear Brain's Inbox, Improve Learning. (2018, August 22). Retrieved from https://news.nationalgeographic.com/news/2010/02/100222-sleep-naps-brain-memories/

National Sleep Foundation (2007). Facts about drowsy driving. Retrieved from http://drowsydriving.org/2014/10/facts-about-drowsy-driving/

National Sleep Foundation (2012). How much sleep do we really need? Retrieved from https://sleepfoundation.org/how-sleep-works/how-much-sleep-do-we-really-need

National Sleep Foundation (2015). Myths and facts about sleep. Retrieved from https://sleepfoundation.org/how-sleep-works/myths-and-facts-about-sleep

Neuroscience News.com 2015). Researchers find missing link between the brain and the immune system. Retrieved from http://neurosciencenews.com/lymphatic-system-brain-neurobiology-2080/

Nursing World (2016). 2011 ANA Health and Safety Survey. Retrieved from http://www.nursingworld.org/2011HealthSurveyResults.aspx

NYU Langone Health / NYU School of Medicine. (2019, April 16). Common sleep myths compromise good sleep and health. *ScienceDaily*. Retrieved from www.sciencedaily.com/releases/2019/04/190416081414.htm

Ohayon, M. M., Mahowald, M. W., Dauvilliers, Y., Krystal, A. D., & Leger, D. (2012). Prevalence and comorbidity of nocturnal wandering in the US adult general population. Neurology,78(20), 1583-1589.

Okun, M. L., Luther, J. F., Wisniewski, S. R., & Wisner, K. L. (2013). Disturbed Sleep and Inflammatory Cytokines in Depressed and Nondepressed Pregnant Women. *Psychosomatic Medicine,75*(7), 670-681.

Paddoc, C. (2018, September 05). Alzheimer's: How does tau disrupt brain cells? Retrieved from https://www.medicalnewstoday.com/articles/322991.php

Paddoc, C. (2015, July 09). Over-the-counter sleep aids linked to dementia. Retrieved from https://www.medicalnewstoday.com/articles/288546.php

Pandi-Perumal, S. R., & Gonfalone, A. A. (2016). Sleep as the new medical frontier: Maintaining proper sleep is critical in space missions. Sleep Science.

Parasomnias & Disruptive Sleep Disorders. (2017, April 22). Retrieved from https://my.clevelandclinic.org/health/diseases/12133-parasomnias-disruptive-sleep-disorders

Park., Y. Yoo, J, Cho, B., Kim, K, Jeong, W & Ha, M. Noise in hospital rooms and sleep disturbance in ... Environ Health Toxicol. 2014;29:e2014006. Epub 2014 Aug 18 Retrieved from https://www.ncbi.nlm.nih.gov/pmc/articles/PMC4152942/

Pearsall, B. (2012). Sleep Disorders, Work Shifts and Officer Wellness. National Institute of Justice, NIJ Journal, 270. Retrieved from http://www.nij.gov/journals/270/pages/officer-wellness.aspx

Person. (2011, May 30). Sleep loss lowers testosterone in healthy young men. Retrieved from https://www.uchicagomedicine.org/forefront/news/2011/may/sleep-loss-lowers-testosterone-in-healthy-young-men

Perrault, A. A., Khani, A., Quairiaux, C., Kompotis, K., Franken, P., Muhlethaler, M., Bayer, L. (2019). Whole-Night Continuous Rocking Entrains Spontaneous Neural Oscillations with Benefits for Sleep and Memory. *Current Biology*.

Philip, P. Taillard, J., Sagaspe, P., Valtat, C., Sanchez-Ortuno, M. et al. (2004). Age, performance and sleep deprivation. Journal of Sleep Research, 13, 105-110.

Pilot asleep, co-pilot on tab, Jet flight drops 5,000 feet (2014, August 14). The Times of India. Retrieved from http://timesofindia.indiatimes.com/india/Pilot-asleep-co-pilot-on-tab-Jet-flight-drops-5000-feet/articleshow/40211580.cms

Poor Sleep in Pregnancy Can Lead to Complications at Birth. (n.d.).

Retrieved from https://www.psychologytoday.com/us/blog/sleep-newzzz/201308/poor-sleep-in-pregnancy-can-lead-complications-birth

Popova, M. (2013). The Art of "Creative Sleep": Stephen King on Writing and Wakeful Dreaming. Brain Pickings. Retrieved from https://www.brainpickings.org/2013/10/14/stephen-king-on-writing-and-creative- sleep/

Ramey, S. L., Perkhounkova, Y., Moon, M., Budde, L., Tseng, H., & Clark, M. K. (2012). The Effect of Work Shift and Sleep Duration on Various Aspects of Police Officers' Health. Workplace Health Workplace Health & Safety, 60(5), 215-222.

Rattenborg, N. C., Voirin, B., Cruz, S. M., Tisdale, R., Dell'Omo, G., Lipp, H., . . . Vyssotski, A. L. (2016, August 03). Evidence that birds sleep in mid-flight. Retrieved from http://www.nature.com/articles/ncomms12468

Reinberg, S. (2015, November 5). Poor Sleep Might Harm Kidneys, Study Suggests. Retrieved from http://www.webmd.com/sleep- disorders/news/20151105/poor-sleep-might-harm-kidneys-study-suggests

Ritter, S. M., Strick, M., Bos, M. W., Baaren, R. B., & Dijksterhuis, A. (2012). Good morning creativity: Task reactivation during sleep enhances beneficial effect of sleep on creative performance. Journal of Sleep Research, 21(6), 643-647.

Roazen, P. (1992). Freud and his followers. New York: Da Capo Press.

Roehrs, T., and Roth, T. Sleep, Sleepiness, and Alcohol Use. *NIAA.* https://pubs.niaaa.nih.gov/publications/arh25-2/101-109.htm

Romero, R., & Badr, M. (2014, January). A role for sleep disorders in pregnancy complications ... Retrieved from http://myspecialist.clinic/uploads/3/4/8/4/34848987/review_sleep_disorderes_and_preganancy_challenges_and_opportunities.pdf

Rosen, L., Whaling, K., Rab, S., Carrier, L., & Cheever, N. (2013). Is Facebook creating "iDisorders"? The link between clinical symptoms of psychiatric disorders and technology use, attitudes and anxiety. Computers in Human Behavior,29(3), 1243-1254.

Samson, D. R., Manus, M. B., Krystal, A. D., Fakir, E., Yu, J. J., & Nunn,

C. L. (2017). Segmented sleep in a nonelectric, small-scale agricultural society in Madagascar. American Journal of Human Biology.

Sandoiu, A. (2019, January 29). Why sleep is the best painkiller. Retrieved from https://www.medicalnewstoday.com/articles/324316.php

Sandoiu, A. How does alcohol affect your sleep. *Medical News Today*, 7 May 2018.

Saul, S. (2006, March 14). Study links Ambien use to unconscious food forays. New York Times. Retrieved from http://www.nytimes.com/2006/03/14/health/14sleep.html?

Sateia, M. J., Buysse, D. J., Krystal, A. D., & Neubauer, D. N. (2017). Adverse Effects of Hypnotic Medications. *Journal of Clinical Sleep Medicine,13*(06), 839-839. doi:10.5664/jcsm.6634

Schabus, M., Griessenberger, H., Gnjezda, M., et al. (2017). Better than sham? A double-blind placebo-controlled neurofeedback study in primary insomnia. Brain, 1-12.

Seligman, M. E. (2002). Authentic happiness: Using the new positive psychology to realize your potential for lasting fulfillment. New York: Free Press.

Seppa, N. (2014, June 10). Daylight saving time linked to heart attacks. Retrieved from https://www.sciencenews.org/article/daylight-saving-time-linked-to-heart-attacks

Sexton, C. E., Storsve, A. B., Walhovd, K. B., Johansen-Berg, H., & Fjell, A. M. (2014). Poor sleep quality is associated with increased cortical atrophy in community-dwelling adults. Neurology,83(11), 967-973.

Sharpless, B. A., & Doghramji, K. (2015). What Are Sleep Paralysis and Isolated Sleep Paralysis? Sleep Paralysis, 1-6.

Sheikh, K. (2016, February 05). Early Bird or Night Owl? It May Be in Your Genes. Retrieved from http://www.livescience.com/53624-morning-person-genetic-influence.html

Shobeiri, F., Khaledi, S., Masoumi, S., & Roshanaei, G. (2016). The effect of music therapy counseling on sleep quality in pregnant women. International J. of Medical Research & Health Sciences, 5, 9S: 408-416.

Sicart, M. (2014). Play matters. Cambridge, MA: MIT.

Siegel, I., & Kryger, M. H. (2016). When sleep is intertwined with myth. Sleep Health, 2(3), 183-184.

Sinha, P. (Sept. 4, 2014). Why do doctors commit suicide? New York Times, Op-Ed. Sleep Hygiene Tips. (n.d.). Retrieved from https://www.mountsinai.org/locations/respiratory-institute/treatments/sleep-disorders/hygiene-tips

Sleep, Learning, and Memory. (n.d.). Retrieved from http://healthysleep.med.harvard.edu/healthy/matters/benefits-of-sleep/learning-memory

Sleep paralysis. (2016, July 2). Retrieved from www.nhs.uk Sleep, Performance, and Public Safety. (n.d.). Retrieved from http://healthysleep.med.harvard.edu/healthy/matters/consequences/sleep-performance-and-public-safety

Sleep Violence: Rare, but Real « Sleep Well. (n.d.). Retrieved from http://blogs.webmd.com/sleep-disorders/2010/04/sleep-violence-rare-but-real.html

Smith, G. (2014, March 27). Sundowning: Late-day confusion. Retrieved February 27, 2016, from http://www.mayoclinic.org/sundowning/expert-answers/faq-20058511

Stem cell specialization observed in the brain. (2015). Neuroscience from Technology Networks. Retrieved from http://www.neuroscientistnews.com/research-news/stem-cell-specialization-observed-brain

Stages of Sleep: The Sleep Cycle – American Sleep Association. (n.d.). Retrieved from https://www.sleepassociation.org/about-sleep/stages-of-sleep/

Stern, P. (2017). Synapse remodeling during sleep. Science,355(6324).

Stutz, J., Eiholzer, R., & Spengler, C. M. (2018). Effects of Evening Exercise on Sleep in Healthy Participants: A Systematic Review and Meta-Analysis. Sports Medicine.

Snowdon, D. (2008). Aging with grace: The nun study and the science of old age: how we can all live longer, healthier and more vital lives. London: Fourth Estate.

Snowdon, D. (2000). The Nun Study - Alzheimer Monterrey. http://www.alzheimermonterrey.com/estudios/estudios/Estudio-Monjas-I.pdf

Stewart-Williams, S. & Podd, J. (2004). The Placebo Effect: Dissolving the Expectancy Versus Conditioning Debate. Psychological Bulletin, Vol.130, No.2, pp.324-340.

Stony Brook University (2015, August 4). Science Daily. Could body posture during sleep affect how your brain clears waste? Retrieved from http://www.sciencedaily.com/releases/2015/08/150804203440.htm

Stromberg, J. (2012, June 26). Experiments Show We Really Can Learn While We Sleep. Retrieved from http://www.smithsonianmag.com/science-nature/experiments-show-we-really-can-learn-while-we-sleep-141518869/

Stromberg, J. (2012, July 23). What Is the Nocebo Effect? http://www.smithsonianmag.com/science-nature/what-is-the-nocebo-effect-5451823/

Suicide Risk and Sleep: What's the Link? Psychiatric Times. (2018, November 20). Retrieved from https://www.psychiatrictimes.com/cme/suicide-risk-and-sleep-whats-link

Tamaki, M., et al. (2016) Night Watch in One Brain Hemisphere during Sleep Associated with the First-Night Effect in Humans. Current Biology 26(9), 1190-1194.

Tamm, S. (2019). A sleep-deprived brain interprets impressions negatively. Retrieved April 8, 2019, from https://ki.se/en/news/a-sleep-deprived-brain-interprets-impressions-negatively

Tau protein. (2019, May 02). Retrieved from https://en.wikipedia.org/wiki/Tau_protein

Tomasulo, D. Proof Positive: Can Heaven Help Us? The Nun Study – Afterlife. (2010, November 03) https://psychcentral.com/blog/archives/2010/10/27/proof-positive-can-heaven-help-us-the-nun-study-afterlife/

Troxel, W. (2018, January 26). Teen-agers need more sleep. That takes good policy as well as good parenting. Retrieved from https://www.usatoday.com/story/opinion/2018/01/26/teen-agers-need-good-parenting-and-good-policy-get-more-sleep-wendy-troxel-column/1065083001/

Tryptophan. (2014, May 9). MedLine Plus. Retrieved from https://www.nlm.nih.gov/medlineplus/ency/article/002332.htm

Trahan, T., Durrant, S. J., Müllensiefen, D., & Williamson, V. J. (n.d.). The music that helps people sleep and the reasons they believe it works: A mixed methods analysis of online survey reports. Retrieved from https://journals.plos.org/plosone/article?id=10.1371/journal.pone.0206531

Tsai, H. J., Kuo, T. B., Lee, G., & Yang, C. C. (2014). Efficacy of paced breathing for insomnia: Enhances vagal activity and improves sleep quality. Psychophysiology,52(3), 388-396. doi:10.1111/psyp.12333

University of Maryland Medical Center, In-depth Patient Education Reports. Insomnia. Retrieved from http://umm.edu/health/medical/reports/articles/insomnia

Understanding and Addressing Sleep Disruptions in Alcohol ... (n.d.). Retrieved from https://www.psychiatrictimes.com/special-reports/understanding-and-addressing-sleep-disruptions-alcohol-use-disorders

University of Rochester Medical Center (2013, October 17). Newsroom. To Sleep, Perchance to Clean. Retrieved from https://www.urmc.rochester.edu/news/story/3956/to-sleep-perchance-to- clean.aspx

University of Rochester Medical Center (2012, August 15). Scientists discover previously unknown cleansing system in brain. Retrieved from https://www.urmc.rochester.edu/news/story/3584/scientists-discover-previously-unknown-cleansing-system-in-brain.aspx

Urrila, A.S., Artiges, E., Massicotte, J., et al. (2017, February 09). Sleep habits, academic performance and the adolescent brain structure. Scientific Reports 7, Article number 41678.

Valham, F., Sahlin, C., Stenlund, H., & Franklin, K. (2012). Ambient temperature and obstructive sleep apnea: Effects of sleep, sleep apnea and morning alertness. Sleep, 35(4), 513-517.

Van Cauter, E., Knutson, K., Leproult, R., & Spiegel, K. (2005). The impact of sleep deprivation on hormones and metabolism. Medscape, Psychiatry & Mental Health. Retrieved from http://www.medscape.org/viewarticle/502825

Van Dam, N & van der Helm, E. (2016, February 16). There's a Proven Link Between Effective Leadership and Getting Enough Sleep. Harvard Business Review, February 16, 2016. Retrieved from https://hbr.org/2016/02/theres-a-proven-link-  between-effective-leadership-and-getting-enough-sleep

Ventricular system. (2017, February 22). Retrieved from https://en.wikipedia.org/wiki/Ventricular_system

Verster, J. C., Taillard, J., Sagaspe, P., Olivier, B., & Philip, P. (2011). Prolonged nocturnal driving can be as dangerous as severe alcohol-impaired driving. Journal of Sleep Research, 20(4), 585-588.

Vivo, L. D., Bellesi, M., Marshall, W., Bushong, E. A., Ellisman, M. H., Tononi, G., & Cirelli, C. (2017). Ultrastructural evidence for synaptic scaling across the wake/sleep cycle. Science,355(6324), 507-510.

Voss, W. (2002). Contributing factors to depressed mood in multiple sclerosis. Archives of Clinical Neuropsychology, 17(2), 103-115.

UW sleep research high-resolution images show how the brain resets during sleep. (n.d.). Retrieved from http://news.wisc.edu/uw-sleep-research-high-resolution-images-show-how-the-brain-resets-during-sleep/

Wagner, U., Gais, S., Haider, H., Verleger, R., & Born, J. (2004). Sleep inspires insight. Nature, 427(6972), 352-355.

Watson, N., Harden, K., Buchwald, D., Vitiello, M., Pack, A. et al. (2014). Sleep duration and depressive symptoms: a gene-environment interaction. Sleep, 37(2), 351- 358.

Webster, M. (2008, May 6). Can you catch up on lost sleep? Scientific American. Retrieved from http://www.scientificamerican.com/article/fact-or-fiction-can-you-catch-up-on-sleep/

Weintraub, K. Catching up on lost sleep (2015, July 24). Well, New York Times.

Wen, T. (2014, April 10). The Ways to Control Dreaming. Retrieved from http://www.theatlantic.com/health/archive/2014/04/the-ways-to-control-dreaming/360032/

West, S. D., Lochmüller, H., Hughes, J., Atalaia, A., Marini-Bettolo, C., Baudouin, S. V., & Anderson, K. N. (2016). Sleepiness and Sleep-related Breathing Disorders in Myotonic Dystrophy and Responses to Treatment: A Prospective Cohort Study. Journal of Neuromuscular Diseases,3(4), 529-537.

Westwood, A. J., Beiser, A., Jain, N., Himali, J. J., Decarli, C., Auerbach, S. H., .Seshadri, S. (2016). Prolonged sleep duration as a marker of early neurodegeneration predicting incident dementia. Neurology.

What Is Beautiful Is Good. (n.d.). Retrieved from 1972. Vol. 24, No. 3, 285-290 http://faculty.uncfsu.edu/tvancantfort/Syllabi/Gresearch/Readings/17Dion.pdf

What is Sleep? Why is it needed? – American Sleep Association. (n.d.). Retrieved from https://www.sleepassociation.org/about-sleep/what-is-sleep/

Whether You're a Lark or a Night Owl, Your Sleeping Habits Say Volumes About Your Health. (n.d.). Retrieved from http://preventdisease.com/news/13/081213_Whether-Your-a-Lark-or-a-Night-Owl-Your-Sleeping-Habits-Say-Volumes-About-Your-Health.shtml

Williams, W. C. (n.d.). The Use of Force--William Carlos Williams (1883-1963). Retrieved from http://bitly.com/2WWnFmH

Williamson, V. (2016, October 23). Why listening to music before bed can beat insomnia. Retrieved from https://www.newsweek.com/music-insomnia-sleep-better-sleep-sleeping-habits-health-wellbeing-scientific-511280

Wilson, C. (n.d.). We've discovered a new type of blood vessel in our bones. Retrieved from https://www.newscientist.com/article/2191282-weve-discovered-a-new-type-of-blood-vessel-in-our-bones/

Winsler, A., Deutsch, A., Verona, R., Payne, P., & Szklo-Coxe, M. (2014, May 13). Sleepless in Fairfax: The Difference One More Hour of ... Retrieved from http://winslerlab.gmu.edu/pubs/WinslerSleep.pdf

Wolf-Meyer, M. J. (2014). Myths of Modern American Sleep: Naturalizing Primordial Sleep, Blaming Technological Distractions, and Pathologizing Children. Science as Culture,24(2), 205-226.

World Health Organization, Road traffic injuries. Key facts, updated October 2015. Retrieved from http://www.who.int/mediacentre/factsheets/fs358/en/

Wołyńczyk-Gmaj D, Różańska-Walędziak A, Ziemka S, Ufnal M, Brzezicka A, Gmaj B, Januszko P, Fudalej S, Czajkowski K, Wojnar M. Insomnia in pregnancy is associated with depressive symptoms and eating at night. *J Clin Sleep Med.*2017;13(10):1171–1176.

Why sleep is important and what happens when you don't get enough. (2004, September 15). Retrieved from http://www.apa.org/topics/sleep/why.aspx

Yang, G., Lai, C. S., Cichon, J., Ma, L., Li, W., & Gan, W. (2014). Sleep promotes branch-specific formation of dendritic spines after learning. Science, 344(6188), 1173-1178.

Young, S. (2013, September 27). Half of British pilots admit to falling asleep in cockpit – survey. Reuters Life, London. Retrieved from http://www.reuters.com/article/us-britain-pilots-sleep-idUSBRE98Q0L820130927

Welsh, J. (2013, October 17). Scientists Have Finally Found The First Real Reason We Need To Sleep. Retrieved from https://www.businessinsider.com/the-first-real-reason-we-need-to-sleep-2013-10.

# The Life Stress Scale

Place a check next to each item that applies to you. Then add up your score.

|  | VALUE |
|---|---|
| Death of spouse | 100 |
| Divorce | 73 |
| Marital Separation | 65 |
| Jail Term | 63 |
| Death of close family member | 63 |
| Personal injury or illness | 53 |
| Marriage | 50 |
| Fired at work | 47 |
| Marital reconciliation | 45 |
| Retirement | 45 |
| Change in health of family member | 44 |
| Pregnancy | 40 |
| Sex difficulties | 39 |
| Gain of a new family member | 39 |
| Business readjustment | 39 |
| Change in financial state | 38 |
| Death of a close friend | 37 |
| Change to a different line of work | 36 |

| Change in number of arguments with spouse | 35 |
| Mortgage over $20,000 | 31 |
| Foreclosure of mortgage or loan | 30 |
| Change in responsibilities at work | 29 |
| Son or daughter leaving home | 29 |
| Trouble with in laws | 29 |
| Outstanding personal achievement | 28 |
| Spouse begins or stop work | 26 |
| Begin or end school | 26 |
| Change in living conditions | 25 |
| Revisions of personal habits | 24 |
| Trouble with boss | 23 |
| Change in work hours or conditions | 20 |
| Change in residence | 20 |
| Change in schools | 20 |
| Change in recreations | 19 |
| Change in church activities | 19 |
| Change in social activities | 19 |
| Mortgage or loan less than $20,000 | 17 |
| Change in sleeping habits | 16 |
| Change in number of family get-togethers | 15 |
| Change in eating habits | 15 |
| Vacation | 13 |
| Christmas approaching | 12 |
| Minor violation of the law | 11 |
| Total | |

*Used with permission of Dr. Richard Rahe*

## The scores

**300 or over** must be carefully considered as being at risk for illness (the immune system is especially vulnerable to stress levels). When stress goes up, your body's ability to maintain your health goes down. The immune system has a direct connection to stress.

**151 – 299** means you may be at moderate risk for illness

**150 or less** is considered a slight risk of illness

Remember, these scores don't predict illness, but they are like road signs in your life telling you that there's a possible dangerous curve ahead and you need to proceed with caution. Not a bad thing to do and, in fact, it's always good to see something that may be coming down the road so that you can take appropriate action.

Now, how about asking yourself a few questions about how you've been feeling lately? This is just to provide you with some additional information about where you might want to make some changes.

| | |
|---|---|
| First, how have you been sleeping? | Number of hours: _____ |
| Have you been having conflicts with anyone? | __ yes ___no |
| Do you find yourself becoming anxious? | ___yes ___ no |
| Do you feel you have little time for yourself? | ___yes ___ no |
| Do you feel you've done a good job as a caregiver? | ___yes __ no |
| Are you feeling depressed? | __ yes ___ no |
| Do you feel trapped in any way? | ___ yes ___no |
| Is a sense of resentfulness taking over you? | ___ yes ___no |

There's no score for these last few questions but in thinking each of them over, you may begin to come in touch with things that are bothering you. If you're not sleeping well, what might be the reason? What about having conflicts with anyone? Is this something new for you and how often is it happening, if it's happening?

What about your level of anxiety? Everyone gets anxious sometime and that's normal because there are things that make all of us anxious. But if you're feeling more anxious than usual, what is the source of that anxiety? Think it over.

Need I add an additional word about allowing yourself the pleasure and restoration you need by sleeping or napping when you can, as much as you can? I'm not advocating that you engage in a life of total leisure here, but I want you to give yourself a break; you deserve it.

I know how hard all of you work at your many roles and each takes something from you, so be sure to recharge those emotional and physical batteries but don't skimp on your sleep..

# Morning-Eveningness Questionnaire

Are you a night owl or an early bird?

## Instructions

Read each question carefully. Answer each question as honestly as possible. Do not go back and check your answers. *Your first response* is usually the most accurate. Circle the number (score) next to the time that applies best to you.

Answer ALL questions.

**1. What time would you get up if you were entirely free to plan your day?**

| Time | Score (please circle) |
| --- | --- |
| 5:00 – 6:29 am | 5 |
| 6:30 – 7:44 am | 4 |
| 7:45 – 9:44 am | 3 |
| 9:45 – 10:59 am | 2 |
| 11:00 – 11:59 am | 1 |
| Midday – 5:00 am | 0 |

2. **What time would you go to bed if you were entirely free to plan your evening?**

| Time | Score |
|---|---|
| 8:00 – 8:59 pm | 5 |
| 9:00 – 10:14 pm | 4 |
| 10:15 pm – 12:29 am | 3 |
| 12:30 – 1:44 am | 2 |
| 1:45 – 2:59 am | 1 |
| 3:00 am – 8:00 pm | 0 |

**Specific time at which you have to get up in the morning? To what extent do you depend on being awakened by an alarm clock?**

| | Score |
|---|---|
| Not at all dependent | 4 |
| Slightly dependent | 3 |
| Fairly dependent | 2 |
| Very dependent | 1 |

3. **How easy do you find it to get up in the morning (when you are not awakened unexpectedly)?**

| | Score |
|---|---|
| Not at all easy | 1 |
| Not very easy | 2 |
| Fairly easy | 3 |
| Very easy | 4 |

4. **How alert do you feel during the first half hour after you wake up in the morning?**

| | Score |
|---|---|
| Not at all alert | 1 |
| Slightly alert | 2 |
| Fairly alert | 3 |
| Very alert | 4 |

5. **How hungry do you feel during the first half-hour after you wake up in the morning?**

|  | Score |
|---|---|
| Not at all hungry | 1 |
| Slightly hungry | 2 |
| Fairly hungry | 3 |
| Very hungry | 4 |

6. **During the first half-hour after you wake up in the morning, how tired do you feel?**

|  | Score |
|---|---|
| Very tired | 1 |
| Fairly tired | 2 |
| Fairly refreshed | 3 |
| Very refreshed | 4 |

7. **If you have no commitment the next day, what time would you go to bed compared to your usual bedtime?**

|  | Score |
|---|---|
| Seldom or never later | 4 |
| Less than one hour later | 3 |
| 1-2 hours later | 2 |
| More than two hours later | 1 |

8. **You have decided to engage in some physical exercise. A friend suggests that you do this for one hour twice a week and the best time for him/her is between 7:00 – 8:00 am. Bearing in mind nothing but your own internal "clock", how do you think you would perform?**

|                              | Score |
| ---------------------------- | ----- |
| Would be in good form        | 4     |
| Would be in reasonable form  | 3     |
| Would find it difficult      | 2     |
| Would find it very difficult | 1     |

9.  **At what time of day do you feel you become tired as a result of need for sleep?**

| Time                    | Score |
| ----------------------- | ----- |
| 8:00 – 8:59 pm          | 5     |
| 9:00 – 10:14            | 4     |
| 10:15 pm – 12:44 am     | 3     |
| 12:45 – 1:59 am         | 2     |
| 2:00 – 3:00 am          | 1     |

10. **You want to be at your peak performance for a test that you know is going to be mentally exhausting and will last for two hours. You are entirely free to plan your day. Considering only your own internal "clock", which ONE of the four testing times would you choose?**

| Time                 | Score |
| -------------------- | ----- |
| 8:00 – 10:00 am      | 4     |
| 11:00 am – 1:00 pm   | 3     |
| 3:00 – 5:00 pm       | 2     |
| 7:00 – 9:00 pm       | 1     |

11. **If you got into bed at 11:00 pm, how tired would you be?**

|                   | Score |
| ----------------- | ----- |
| Not at all tired  | 1     |
| A little tired    | 2     |
| Fairly tired      | 3     |
| Very tired        | 4     |

12. **For some reason, you have gone to bed several hours later than usual, but there is no need to get up at any particular time the next morning. Which ONE of the following are you most likely to do?**

|  | Score |
|---|---|
| Will wake up at usual time, but will NOT fall back asleep | 4 |
| Will wake up at usual time and will doze thereafter | 3 |
| Will wake up at usual time but will fall asleep again | 2 |
| Will NOT wake up until later than usual | 1 |

13. **One night you have to remain awake between 4:00 – 6:00 am in order to carry out a night watch. You have no commitments the next day. Which ONE of the alternatives will suite you best?**

|  | Score |
|---|---|
| Would NOT go to bed until watch was over | 1 |
| Would take a nap before and sleep after | 2 |
| Would take a good sleep before and nap after | 3 |
| Would sleep only before watch | 4 |

14. **You have to do two hours of hard physical work. You are entirely free to plan your day and considering only your own internal "clock" which ONE of the following times would you choose?**

| Time | Score |
|---|---|
| 8:00 – 10:00 am | 4 |
| 11:00 am – 1:00 pm | 3 |
| 3:00 – 5:00 pm | 2 |
| 7:00 – 9:00 pm | 1 |

15. **You have decided to engage in hard physical exercise. A friend suggests that you do this for one hour twice a week and the best time for him/her is between 10:00 – 11:00 pm. Bearing in mind nothing**

else but your own internal "clock", how well do you think you would perform?

|  | Score |
|---|---|
| Would be in good form | 4 |
| Would be in reasonable form | 3 |
| Would find it difficult | 2 |
| Would find it very difficult | 1 |

16. **Suppose that you can choose your school hours. Assume that you went to school for five hours per day and that school was interesting and enjoyable. Which five consecutive hours would you select?**

|  | Score |
|---|---|
| 5 hours starting between 4:00 – 7:59 am | 5 |
| 5 hours starting between 8:00 – 8:59 am | 4 |
| 5 hours starting between 9:00 am – 1:59 pm | 3 |
| 5 hours starting between 2:00 – 4:59 pm | 2 |
| 5 hours starting between 5:00 pm – 3:59 am | 1 |

17. **At what time of the day do you think that you reach your "feeling best" peak?**

| Time | Score |
|---|---|
| 5:00 – 7:59 am | 5 |
| 8:00 – 9:59 am | 4 |
| 10:00 am – 4:59 pm | 3 |
| 5:00 – 9:59 pm | 2 |
| 10:00 pm – 4:59 am | 1 |

18. **One hears about "morning" and "evening" types of people. Which ONE of these types do you consider yourself to be?**

|  | **Score** |
|---|---|
| Definitely a "morning" type | 6 |
| Rather more a "morning" type than an "evening" type | 4 |
| Rather more an "evening" type than a "morning" type | 2 |
| Definitely an "evening" type | 0 |

## Scoring

Add up the score for all 19 questions and enter it in the box below:

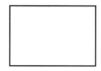

Scores can range from 16-86. **Scores of 41 and below indicate "evening types". Scores of 59 and above indicate "morning types".** Scores between 42 and 58 indicate "intermediate types".

| 16-30 | 31-41 | 42-58 | 59-69 | 70-86 |
|---|---|---|---|---|
| Definite Evening | Moderate Evening | Intermediate | Moderate Morning | Definite Morning |

So what if you are an evening type, yet have to get up early to go to school? The good news is that you **can re-train your body clock** to fit with the times you need to go to sleep and wake up.

*Used with permission and prepared by Dr. Sarah Biggs, The Ritchie Centre, Monash University, Australia 2015. Source: Horne JA and Östberg O. (1976) A self-assessment questionnaire to determine morning-ness-eveningness in human circadian rhythms. International Journal of Chronobiology. 4:97-100.*

# The Insomnia Severity Index

Please rate the CURRENT (i.e. LAST 2 WEEKS) SEVERITY of your insomnia problem(s).

| Insomnia problem | None | Mild | Moderate | Severe | Very severe |
|---|---|---|---|---|---|
| 1. Difficulty falling asleep | 0 | 1 | 2 | 3 | 4 |
| 2. Difficulty staying asleep | 0 | 1 | 2 | 3 | 4 |
| 3. Problem waking up too early | 0 | 1 | 2 | 3 | 4 |

**4. How SATISFIED/DISSATISFIED are you with your CURRENT sleep pattern?**

| Very Satisfied | Satisfied | Moderately Satisfied | Dissatisfied | Very Dissatisfied |
|---|---|---|---|---|
| 0 | 1 | 2 | 3 | 4 |

**5. How NOTICEABLE to others do you think your sleep problem is in terms of impairing the quality of your life?**

| Not at all Noticeable | A Little | Somewhat | Much | Very Much Noticeable |
|---|---|---|---|---|
| 0 | 1 | 2 | 3 | 4 |

**6. How WORRIED/DISTRESSED are you about your current sleep problem?**

| Not at all Worried | A Little | Somewhat | Much | Very Much Worried |
|---|---|---|---|---|
| 0 | 1 | 2 | 3 | 4 |

**7. To what extent do you consider your sleep problem to INTERFERE with your daily functioning (e.g. daytime fatigue, mood, ability to function https://nym.ag/2Lxe0m0at work/daily chores, concentration, memory, mood, etc.) CURRENTLY?**

| Not at all Interfering | A Little | Somewhat | Much | Very Much Interfering |
|---|---|---|---|---|
| 0 | 1 | 2 | 3 | 4 |

**Guidelines for Scoring/Interpretation:**
Add the scores for all seven items' questions = _____your total score

Total score categories:
0-7 = No clinically significant insomnia
8-14 = Subthreshold insomnia
15-21 = Clinical insomnia (moderate severity)
22-28 = Clinical insomnia (severe)

**Print out your completed Insomnia Severity Index, along with the Guidelines for Scoring/Interpretation, to show to your healthcare provider.**

*Used with permission from Charles M. Morin, Ph.D., Université Laval*

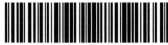
51292584R00125

Made in the USA
Middletown, DE
01 July 2019